Lightbody Activation and Psychic Surgery

Lightbody Activation and Psychic Surgery

Lance Carter

Lightbody Activation and Psychic Surgery

Copyright © 2008 by Lance Carlyle Carter

ISBN 978-1-935057-00-0

Library of Congress Control Number: 2008908079

First Edition

Published by LightCorps™ www.lightcorps.com
Please visit www.lightbodyactivation.com
Lance Carter   www.lancecarter.com
Saratoga, California 95070
Distributed by Amazon.com and other booksellers.

DISCLAIMER

Warning: The goal of this book is to provide information about lightbody activation and psychic surgery. The author is not a doctor. The information contained herein is only the personal opinion of the author. In no way is it to be considered medical advice, which should be obtained from a physician or licensed health care practitioner. This information is not meant to treat, diagnose, cure, or prevent any disease or illness. Consult with your physician or health care specialist before you begin a change in lifestyle that may effect your health. In no event shall the author be liable to you or anyone else for decisions you make. You are responsible for any loss or damage caused directly or indirectly by your using this information and the actions you take. Errors in content may appear although the author has made efforts to correct them. Reliance on this information is solely at your own risk. Reading this book constitutes your voluntary acceptance of the terms and conditions of this medical disclaimer. The information provided herein is incomplete and unproven by modern medical practice and can only serve to educate and entertain.

Dedication

To my parents Delphine and Cornelius

And to...

Dolfina
Jodell Yvonne Bumatay
Arneldo Bumatay
Feline Bumatay Viloria
Yvonne

The Ilokano lineage and the Filipino people.
The ayurvedic healing lineage of India.

The psychic healers of the Philippines and Brazil.
To the healers of all peoples of the world who have struggled to preserve their cultures and traditions and who still practice the ancient healing ways of their ancestors.

Marialyce Caudillo

Father Charles L. Moore

The Father, The Son, and The Holy Spirit

Archangel Gabriel

The White Unicorn

Metatron and Paracelsus

Our Lady of Hope

Acknowledgments

Thanks to Maria Celado for editing the manuscript. Thanks to Geoff Sylvester for help with the graphics. Thanks to Una Hellich White, Ph.D. and Katrina Guglielmelli for help with the audio transcriptions. Thanks to Marialyce Caudillo and Ilima James for reading the manuscript. Thanks to Barbara Deutsch for proofreading the manuscript.

Thanks to Jodell Bumatay, founder and director of the *DOLFINA Ministry of Lucidity,* for reading the manuscript and making many valuable suggestions. For more information about the concepts of lightbody and psychic surgery presented here, please refer to *A Travel Guide to the Other Side For Gatekeepers of Death & Rebirth,* a book by Jodell Yvonne Bumatay. Please visit www.dolfina.org or write to Dolfina of AIWP, P.O.B. 594, Santa Cruz, CA 95061 for information about advanced psychic training.

I acknowledge Jodell Yvonne Bumatay as my master teacher in the psychic surgeon tradition. I also acknowledge the lightspirits of Dolfina, Arneldo Bumatay, Feline Bumatay Viloria and Yvonne as master teachers. I am grateful to the Ilokano tribal lineage across the ages who assisted in my education. Thanks to the grandmothers and grandfathers.

Thanks to Lord Vishnu for his translation of the text that began this healing tradition thousands of years ago.

Thanks to the healers and Psychic Surgeons of all time.

Thanks to Pearl Dorris of Mount Shasta for sharing the wisdom of lightbody and angels.

Thanks to Saint Germain for training me in Mount Shasta.

Thanks to Father Charles L. Moore for counsel about my visions of apparitions of the Blessed Mother Mary.

Thanks to the Blessed Mother Mary, Our Lady of Hope, for teaching me lightbody technology. Hail Mary!

About the Author

Lance Carter, CID is a Certified Interconnect Designer in the field of electronics packaging design.

Lance was born on October 10, 1950 at 8:16 A.M. in San Francisco, California. Lance was introduced to crystal gazing, Ouija board, automatic writing, tarot, and astrology as a child.

Lance had his chart read by Carroll Righter, "The Astrologer to the Stars". Lance corresponded and conversed with Marc Edmund Jones, Ph.D., "The Dean of American Astrology."

Lance later became an astrologer for newspapers, radio, and the Internet. He has authored articles and taught classes.

Lance has produced and directed open microphone and interview television shows and hosted the SHIFT Lecture Series.

Lance attended talks by Pearl Dorris of Mount Shasta.

Lance studied decipherment with Hugh A. Moran, Ph.D.

Lance studied zen meditation with master Kobin Chino.

Lance studied kundalini yoga and other yoga practices.

Lance studied the Keys of Enoch with J.J. Hurtak, Ph.D.

Lance studied history with Father Charles L. Moore.

Lance studied with the Dolfina Ministry of Lucidity.

Lance was trained in angelic activation by Mother Mary.

Lance channels Paracelsus, the Renaissance surgeon.

Lance also channels the White Unicorn and Metatron.

Please visit www.astromancy.com for astromancy reports.

Please visit www.ladyofhope.net for more information about apparitions of Mother Mary and the Garabandal Warning.

Please visit www.lancecarter.com to link to Lance's articles.

Lance Carlyle Carter offers training in lightbody activation, crystal technology, and psychic ability at seminars, workshops, retreats, and events. Please visit www.lightbodyactivation.com for more information about lightbody activation and other topics.

Please visit www.lightcorps.com for Lance's publications.

Preface

Much of this book is a compilation of channeled teachings of Paracelsus that I dictated in 2007 and then had transcribed and edited. The surgeon Paracelsus is not a ghostwriter. The text is presented as close to verbatim as possible, although instances of archaic English were updated. No attempt has been made to remove repetitious statements or concepts. Much of this book was channeled at night. Usually I was roused out of my sleep to channel. The dictations would begin a few seconds after I turned on the voice recorder and I immediately fell asleep again when they ended. Some nights would involve several dictations.

This information herein is a contribution of many lightbody lineages and the entire lightbody community, which exists in the lightrealm. The lightrealm is also known as the lightworld or the spiritworld. Lightspirits were instrumental in organizing the ideas and retrieving specific topics for dictation. The healing traditions described herein are part of a wider school of thinking that connected the peoples of the ancient world through calendars, math, writing systems, languages, and science. This knowledge still exists in various forms in many indigenous traditions.

My role as the channel sometimes gave me an inside look at the libraries of information that were accessed for these dictations. These libraries sometimes appeared to float in front of me. Blocks of information would break off and come rushing at me and then illuminate me just at the moment I needed to say what that block of information was about. I translated the images and ideas into my own words as I dictated.

References to classes I have taught in the past and personal experiences are sometimes included. Also included are chapters with messages from the White Unicorn, the Ambassador Crystal, and the Blessed Mother Mary.

Lance Carter, aka Paracelsus

Contents

The Lightbody Realm

The lightbody realm is a place that is so different from our ordinary reality that our ordinary consciousness may not comprehend it or remember it very well. In some cases it is totally forgotten. Experiences in the lightbody world are very special, enlightening, elucidating, and vivid. These experiences are often deemed as religious, sacred, mystical and visionary. These visionary phenomena have often and usually been characteristic of young children, females, and some males.

There is also the strange phenomenon that occurs around children. Their closeness to these other worlds may enable some of them to travel within these other worlds as well. The ability of people to see the lightworld can be learned as a child. If lightbody is learned as a child, it is not so strange to learn as an adult.

How do you analyze lightbody? Understand that lightbody is reality. Lightbody is not normally visible to everyone. It is invisible to most people. Those who are trained to see lightbody have a whole new world of lightbody to live in and experience. The lightrealm is this world's other dimension that we are capable of entering, experiencing, and enjoying. We have the ability to travel within the lightbody world, which is our world as well.

There are other spectra of reality in the lightrealm as we travel from the material realm to other more ethereal realms without having actual words to describe them, though there are words in many knowledge systems that describe the levels of light. The lightbody realm co-exists in this realm. It is sometimes called the fourth dimension. But this lightbody realm, whatever dimension it might be called, is probably not a dimension that we can attribute to any number such as one, two, three, four, or five. There might be good systems for doing that.

These lightrealms are known by their frequency, magnitude, and actual disturbances in the nothingness of the void of reality.

Lightbody Technology

Lightbody technology is going to change the future of the world because the future is going to be very closely connected to the development of lightbody technology. In our future on our world, people all around the world will spontaneously know how to do lightbody healing.

Lightbody healing is a talent of everybody on earth. Every human on earth has this talent and it is a characteristic of animals, plants, and rocks. The healing characteristic of lightbody guides the physical body to heal and to become whole. In the future the knowledge of lightbody will become universal, or nearly so.

Lightbody as a way of life has existed for thousands of years in many cultures. Lightbody knowledge, practices, and traditions enhance the individual, family, clan, tribe, and nation to live and to become healthy and whole. In the future this knowledge will become commonplace because it is already within the birthright and within the genome or genes of all humans.

Having this connection to the lightbody means that people can heal and can be healed. This tradition was actually begun by Lord Vishnu in his translation of a particular text, but the tradition had roots all around the world. Lightbody healing is simply a natural occurrence of life.

The use of lightbody healing will become widespread in India, Asia, and other outlying areas. It may spread to the Moslem world as well. The Christian world has already experienced this phenomenon in the Philippines and Brazil. This type of lightbody healing will become more widespread.

This is an evangelical movement, yet it is nondenominational. Christians, Moslems, Jews, Buddhists, Jains, and animists can do this lightbody healing. All of the tribal indigenous people have knowledge of lightbody healing technology. What will be different in the future is that because of the coordination of lightbody technicians and lightbody workers there will be an activation of lightbody healing across the planet.

This means that all having connection to various lightbody connective networks will be activated in certain ways and forms. Usually that activation is what is called a third eye activation of consciousness. It may involve chakra or aura activations. Activations of spirit may occur in other realms, such as emotional, mental, physical, and even environmental. These changes are necessary to accommodate the lightbody future of humanity, the animals, spirits, and the planet.

As a whole we have our future ahead of us as lightbodies. There are certain things and techniques that we can do to fulfill our lightbody destiny. Lightbody destiny is part of the lightbody shape or form. It is the flow or path that the lightbody takes through space and time. Lightbody destiny is at times influenced by decisions, by mortal decisions, by each and everybody wanting to make their own choices. This is good because it helps the furtherance of humanity and life.

On another lightbody level, we go on through lives, we go on through time, we go on through space, and we go on through mind. This lightbody connectivity that we have to everybody means that in our spirit, which is lightbody, we are connected to everybody. In our connectivity we are all harmonized by the resonance of this lightbody activation.

Being interested in studying lightbody technology is a noble pursuit, but what does technology have to do with lightbody? Technology provides the means to use the lightbody to enjoy the experience of the lightbody universe.

Lightbody technology is a form of technology based on using the lightbody. The lightbody consists of a body of energy, which is termed to be light although it has many characteristics and attributes. The characteristics and attributes of the lightbody correspond to the physical body of the person. The lightbody is usually identified with the physical body. For instance, I have a lightbody. You have a lightbody. We all have lightbodies.

Where is the lightbody? In most people the lightbody is within the body and it is often termed as part of the aura and is not extended outside the body. It is usually within the body. It is not what one would term to be the aura, which is a physical manifestation of the physical body.

The lightbody itself resembles the body in most instances, although it can be changed to other forms through the use of willpower. The person in the physical body usually controls their own lightbody. If lightbodies are under manipulation or attack, then they might take on different forms as well. It is best that people maintain their own lightbody integrity so that it does not get distorted. It might lose the characteristics of identity and identification with the actual physical body of the person.

Many know that we have a soul. Some call it a spirit. We definitely have minds and emotions. How about it? Is our lightbody real, or is it a figment of the imagination? Too many people have seen the lightbody and its manifestation to ignore it. We will assume that it is something.

The lightbody being is composed of many types of energy and may be seen on many levels. It has many classifications and attributes. Some of these attributes are seen in the aura, which can extend out from the body a few inches to nearly fifty feet. There are various shells of the aura that extend out from the physical body. This is all part of the lightbody because the lightbody is composed of many different parts of the body and it is all integrated. The lightbody is able to be in various forms.

The physical form is the densest form and the other auric forms that form around the physical form are other forms of the lightbody. The lightbody that is within the body is an example of the perfect structure of the body and it is the example that is set for health, for maintaining health, and for attaining health. Lightbody health is a most important matter for survival for the physical body. Resonance and harmony with one's lightbody is essential for physical health in this system of correspondence. Your lightbody pattern is the pattern that gives your lightbody the ability to be healed and to heal the physical body. That means that if the healing force of a lightbody worker is applied to a disease of a physical body, there is the possibility that the lightbody would be able to reshape the physical body according to the lightbody blueprint. When the psychic surgery or lightbody surgery is occurring, the actual shape and form of the real lightbody is being reimprinted into the physical body at that time. That is done by the action of the lightbody worker, the lightbody physician, and the lightbody surgeon.

Lightbodies are like angels and they are angels. Your lightbody is your angel. You are an angel. We are angels all together in our world we share, in our lightbodies, in our physical bodies, in our mental bodies, in our emotional bodies, and in all of our other auric bodies that emanate and come from the spirit that occupies the physical body.

Lightbody is the body that governs the physical body. Lightbody is the imaginative power. Lightbody is beyond imagination. Lightbody is the structure. Lightbody is the form. Lightbody makes it all happen. Lightbody is the mind. Lightbody is the imagination. Lightbody is the structure and the form. Lightbody makes our life possible. Lightbody is our life because we are life. Lifebody is the living body. Lifebody and lightbody combine and make our physical body reality. What we become is our lightbody. My lightbody is in me and your lightbody is in you.

The lightbody is the blueprint, and the difference between the lightbody and the physical body is evident to the psychic surgeon. If the physical body is ailing, it is not following its pattern. It is not following its blueprint. It is not following its identity. It is not following its path. Injuries, accidents or different circumstances that the body was not meant to have may have diverted it somehow. Other things could have damaged the body, the emotions, or psychology of the being.

The ideas that you have about what you want to be in your lightbody, and the lightbody missions that you strive to do, and your goals in lightbody living, can be achieved by following the blueprint of your lightbody life. Lightbody life is something you were born with. It is like your genes, but it is the blueprint of your lightbody. Your lightbody is an amalgamation of your life and light and your life in love. You attain what you strive for because you are filled with life and light. In that, you are in the flow.

To travel in lightbody means to know the dimensions of the lightbody realm. That means knowing the dimensions of time and space, matter and antimatter, and other forms of measurement used on earth. These concepts are connected through what we all know as math, science, physics and other forms of those. There are indigenous forms of knowledge that have similar concepts that are analogous to these modern scientific concepts.

The ability of primitive peoples to know these concepts is understandable if one can see that they have connection to a great body of knowledge that transcends the scientific knowledge of today. If we can respect the ancients as being holders of certain technologies that are still beyond our comprehension then possibly we might learn from them.

Learning from primitive peoples means that we must take steps in our self-development that allow us to become greater than what we are, though that means maybe becoming a little more primitive than we now are. That might mean giving up a little of the time one spends doing this or that, to doing something else to attain lightbody harmony by doing lightbody work on their lightbody mission.

Lightbody synchronicity with the physical body, the mental body, the emotional body, and the auric bodies is a matter of learning coordination. Lightbodies are identifiable by the various attributes and significances of the spirit occupying the physical body. The significances depend on the exact consequence their influence has on the other bodies in the equation or procedure. Coordination is learned through experience and training. This connection goes beyond simple linear kinds of connection. It is a multidimensional connection. Lightbody connection is a multidimensional connection. If it is between two people, a lightbody connection can manifest as a resonance between chakras that has an effect between the people. One person or the other person might activate that effect through chakra resonance.

There is also the aura effect caused by the emanations of the aura from the body. The different levels of the aura might be affected by the aura of another person. Lightbody manipulation of various other bodies is a matter of manipulating those various bodies through mental manipulation of lightbody forms.

The lightbody uses the tools of lightbodies to perform various actions in the universe, including healings, surgeries, and miraculous events. Lightbodies are entitled to perform miracles on occasion depending on the necessity. Necessities are going to become much more important in the future as time draws near.

The spirits that occupy space and time are lightbody spirits and they have the right to be lightbody spirits. As lightbody spirits ourselves we have the right to be ourselves. We have the right to live in our lightbodies whether they are independent lightbodies, or lightbodies in physical bodies, which we as humans enjoy.

If one is fortunate enough to live in a physical body, one has won the lightbody experience of a lifetime. As a lightbody in a physical body, one has to take all precautions to safeguard the physical body from harm. Learn to be physically correct about what you do so that you are not in harm's way and are able to fully do your duties.

Lightbody Technician

The lightbody technician is a person that uses lightbody technology to accomplish certain feats or facets of their lightbody training or their lightbody mission. The lightbody worker is a technician. A lightbody technician is a person that can use their skills in the lightbody world to effect change in the lightbody world and possibly in the physical world. The lightbody worker uses certain procedures that have certain parameters whether one's aim is to help a patient or to enlighten. A person that wants information might come to the lightreader who can read the aura, chakras, the lightbody being, and give information to that person.

The lightbody worker should receive training in lightbody healing and lightbody technology that allows lightbody manifestation. This includes communicating with and informing the being of their physical, mental, emotional, or lightbody conditions among a few, and to diagnose problems, and possibly offer solutions. As a part of a lightbody culture, these things become evident to people that are around other lightworkers. Within a family group where people are aware of lightbody, when people are ill in that family or otherwise ill disposed, they are seen sooner in that condition and there can be lightbody healing that can occur with the help of the family at that time.

In the primitive or indigenous forms of using lightbody, it is a form of survival, of mutual self-support, and of continuance of the tradition of that particular race, that lineage, that family, that clan, or nation. This lightbody tradition extends across the world.

In most lightbody traditions the lightbody technician is able to use their ability to effect change by going through various exercises that give the lightbody worker more control. That is what the lightbody worker is actually learning when they are apprenticing and taking classes. They should have an idea about what they are trying to control, what they are getting into control, and why they are learning that control.

That kind of control comes through disciplines such as yoga, concentration, meditation, prayer, dedication, and devotion. These forms of worship and religious practice can activate the lightbody perception in an individual and give them the ability to see other people's lightbodies or to feel those lightbodies and receive information from those lightbodies.

Being a lightbody is actually fun and easy and it is a practice that anybody can do. There are some people that do it naturally. They are doing it naturally without actually calling it lightbody. There are many names for this lightbody love.

It is actually a form of living. It is being in the world and having a connection to the world and having connection to each other through our body, through our mind possibly, and through presence. If we are in close proximity to another's aura, there could be aura interaction. The aura only extends so far, but the lightbody can extend quite far and into any time.

It is the lightbody that is doing much of the work that a light-body worker does, although they must master the skills of using their chakras, kundalini, aura, and presence to actually effect change in the lightbody world.

Being a lightbody person and having the lightbody world so close, one is actually in the presence of many who are enjoying lightbody reality. As more people enjoy lightbody reality it will be easier for others to progress or naturally become lightbody active. A lightbody person is able to extend themselves out of themselves. This may seem strange at first and most people may not imagine they can do it. You are more than you think you are. You can extend your lightbody out of your physical body. Your lightbody can do things that are quite creative.

It is through lightbody manipulation that the healing in psy-chic surgery can be done as well as other forms of manipulation of the lightbody bodies, entities, worlds, vibrations, circumstances, and possibly events. Lightbody workers extend through many circumstances, times, and needs. This is good work. It is work that helps people and helps the person that helps others. It is generally an uplifting practice. Lightbody is advocated by the world's religions in their own particular manner usually in reference to the lightbody masters whom they revere such as saints.

The pursuit of lightbody technology is upon the premise that one can learn to do something that most people do not know about. Using lightbody technology enables a person to do things that are unavailable to those uneducated in lightbody technology. In the beginning the lightbody technologist or lightbody worker has to learn how to use the lightbody in ways that are unusual and involve imaginative powers. Lightworkers can travel from one realm to another with ease as they learn the lightbody skills.

There is a lightbody technology that allows the lightbody technician to do things with their hands that are not in the scope of actual medical instruments. This means that they can shape the form of their instruments according to their imagination. Tools do not have to be right-angled or curved. They do not have to be sharp or have any traditional kinds of form. They have forms that can be used in manifesting the actual healing process.

The healer has an intuitive grasp of what the lightbody needs in the physical body. The lightbody will talk to the lightbody technician. The lightbody will give information to the lightbody physician about what the physical body of the patient requires. In traditional medicine the lightbody spoke to the psychic physician, spoke to the healer, and spoke to the shaman.

Imagine the lightbody extending out, such as out of your hand. Imagine your lightbody hand extending out of your physical hand. Imagine your lightbody leg extending out of your physical leg. Imagine your lightbody appearing outside of your physical body. See your lightbody. You may see your lightbody as a shimmering kind of body. Maybe it is just light. You may see nothing unusual. Maybe there is too much light in the room.

There are many reasons to see a lightbody or not see a lightbody. In most cases your lightbody will not want to step out of your physical body for fear of getting lost in space. You and your lightbody must remain united while you are alive. When the lightbody travels, it must have close contact with the body or it won't want to leave. Why would you want to leave your physical body if you are a lightbody? There are reasons to go to places where most people would not go or could not go.

Lightbody technology involves setting up parameters in your experience so that what you visualize is of a certain format and follows certain conventions. The visualization skills of the lightbody worker are paramount in enabling the lightbody worker to do the work. The lightbody worker must use these lightbody skills, which are primarily in the imaginative or visual area. The lightbody worker must learn to imagine, visualize, and manifest.

These are the characteristics of the lightbody worker. Seeing that they have ability at this will lead them to find their own finesse, talent, and power of lightbody manifestation. In the beginning it involves focusing the mind and the mind's eye in the use of the imagination in the creation of the lightbody reality wanted. As an apprentice learns lightbody technology, they must take into account that what they are seeing is only a small part.

The biggest challenge for the apprentice in this work is maintaining concentration. The difficulty in maintaining concentration when under attack from sources that might distract your attention is so great that practicing lightbody lightwork is one of the most difficult things that one will be challenged with. It is necessary not only to learn to think in one manner, or one routine, or one approach, but to approach thinking on a multilevel, multilayer and multimanner, meaning multidimensional thinking. Multidimensional thinking is required in lightbody technology. The attributes of working in lightbody are multidimensional.

The parameters that are laid out are limitations so that the lightbody student or lightbody apprentice is not lost in the vast lightbody technology. Following certain procedures to attain higher levels of consciousness is within the scope of various religions that allow a higher consciousness to be reached. There is a much higher teaching offered to the lightworker and to the priests and priestesses of various religious practices in their inner circles.

The lightbody technology has many varied forms across the world. It is natural technology. It is ingrained in us to know this technology. It is part of our being to know lightbody technology and to be lightbody workers in our own ways. Lightbody technology is an amazing concept. It allows the person or practitioner to get into an empowering consciousness. It can empower that individual and it can empower other individuals as well.

In the lightbody world, the lightbody worker has to think in a much grander scale to use the technology of this thinking to visualize great things. This sometimes takes coaching by the master of lightbody technology to show the student how to think in lightbody terms using the terminology of lightbody. The student can learn the actual manifestation of lightbody devices, lightbody objects, and other lightbody manifestations through the will, visualization, and imaginative abilities.

What occurs is that if the apprentice learns these kinds of skills then they can work in the lightbody world. They have only a limited access to what can be done. That is why there is always room for the lightbody apprentice, when they become a master, to learn other parts of the lightbody technology, because it is so vast.

There are many skills and professions in the lightbody world. The lightbody technology and the lightbody potentialities are so great that any individual could not master them unless they had quite a long time. That is what lightbody technology is about. It is about a long time. It is about seeing into a long time, into the future and into the past. It is about seeing across minds in time, across minds in our own world, and the worlds to come. It is about seeing into the real worlds around us. It is about seeing into parallel worlds, into parallel dimensions, and universes.

Lightbody Manifestation

The lightbody worker has the potential to manifest change in various places with the permissions and powers that they are granted through their lightbody training. The physical body is the best place to start manifesting lightbody energy. The lightbody energy is part of the physical being, yet it can extend out. The auric energy can extend nearly fifty feet out of the physical body for a strong aura, but the lightbody can go across the universe.

Lightbody manifestation is an attribute of being alive and being human, or being an animal, or an inanimate object. Objects and entities that exist throughout the galaxies and the universe have lightbodies. Most of the time these lightbodies resemble the physical bodies they inhabit.

The construction of the lightbody is usually identical in appearance to the physical body, but the lightbody has character-istics that might be called special attributes or enhancements to the regular body. These enhancements are the ability to use the lightbody in manners that the physical body cannot be used by going places the physical body cannot go, by doing things the physical body is not strong enough, or small enough, or big enough to do.

The things available as tools to the lightbody worker are enhanced by knowledge. The teaching mechanism in lightbody education is the most important part. The controlled manifesta-tion of lightbody energies is only possible by knowing exactly how to use the lightbody and the lightbody attributes.

Entities that assume their lightbodies are in realms where they have other potentials or abilities. They can affect different dimensions of reality, alternate or parallel worlds, and alternate universes. These realities are all somehow co-existent, yet they merge at different nexus points, which are connected by con-sciousness or controlled by mind, consciousness, and will.

13

The aspirant, student or apprentice would need to use the tools of concentration and discipline long enough to effect changes in the lightworld and therefore to effect changes in the real world. Novice and neophyte practitioners of lightbody have limited capabilities to cause change because of their own ignorance. The best they might do in the real world is to share knowledge and experience. To talk about these things in the real world is supportive.

As a lightbody apprentice learns how to manifest lightbody skills, they are becoming more educated, more experienced, and becoming more empowered. These three E's are the triangle of lightbody. In the forward progress of a lightbody education, the student would at first be led along paths of knowledge so that they can learn exactly what is the lightbody world and all the things they can do in their lightbody. Becoming enlightened is the next step.

Lightbody means that the person has consciousness of their physical body, their lightbody, and consciousness of other beings. Lightbodies have consciousness of all of what they are responsible for in the moment and can maintain their concentration on that at the moment. Having lightbody consciousness allows the master or apprentice to manifest experiences, visions, and other phenomena in the lightbody realm that have various coincident properties with reality.

People that are experienced in seeing lightbody phenomena can experience different realities all at the same time. The normal world and a vision of a lightbody entity appearing at the same time is usually the case. When a lightbody appears, it often appears as a translucent or transparent being.

This lightbeing has certain properties that are part of being in the lightworld. The vibration and the intensity of the experience of the viewer are based on the viewer's ability and the lightbody's intention. How much energy is a lightbody going to put into

14

physical world manifestation for the aspirant to see such as in a vision and to be heard clairaudibly?

What often occurs in these phenomena is a consciousness change. The individual aspirant in this study experiences varied phenomena that can change them in many ways. How much does a lightbody manifest in a vision? That is up to the lightbody. Because of lightbody manifestation characteristics, the body of an observer may be affected by radiation and may undergo various physical changes.

These changes may be good or they may be bad depending on the technology used by the visiting lightbeings. There are many forms of lightbeings and many varied technologies, so there is a special difficulty in identifying good and bad technologies and their radiation emissions.

It is a rule of thumb that the individual apprentice has to learn from the master what energies and vibrations are acceptable and what are known hazardous energies. The apprentice learns about the problems and challenges that a lightbody worker would encounter in normal lightworld experience. In the entire lightbody education, one is seeing not only the good, but also the bad. Lightbody is pursued as a phenomenon of religious experience by many religions and practices. In Christianity the religious experience is usually manifested as visions of saints, of Jesus, of Mother Mary, of angels, and the like.

All of these have significance in the lightbody realm and they have an impact on religion. Various religions have their own lightbody beings, entities, and icons as we have come to know them. Lightbody technology is not any particular culture's birthright. It is such a complex technology that it takes a dedicated apprentice to know even a small part of the lightbody technology.

Lightbody technology empowers the apprentice to become a master in their own environment and to effect change within their family, family group, extended family, friends, community, and possibly their tribe, nation and culture. All of these enlightening things can emanate from the apprentice, master, or experiencer of lightbody.

Lightbody education is good for teaching about what to look for when experiencing lightbody phenomena. There are various mystical signs that appear and these are catalogued in religious literatures. Various phenomena such as shimmering light, doorways, windows, and other mysterious phenomena appear as gateways or portals to other worlds, places, and times.

These are the portals that the lightbody worker is interested in. One is interested in not only going through portals, but in creating them, because one does not want to go somewhere where one cannot get back from. The lightbody worker has to recognize these portals, see who and what is on the other side, and not just jump through. One cannot know what is waiting if one has not looked thoroughly.

Creating your own lightbody portals and portals through space and time is done by using the ability to change oneself in space and time, while maintaining contact with the physical body through the lightbody connection. The difficulty and the problem with lightbody adventure is that it has real consequences. If one makes a big mistake, one might end up in heaven with all those other lightbodies, or down below and who wants to go there?

All of our religions have a handle on lightbody technology. It is used to give people within the faith the ability to cope with reality. The lightbody has an ability to be soothing and to comfort the physical. It can make the physical more healthy and alive because it is the live part of the body. It is what we might consider the soul or the spirit. It is more than the intelligence. It is the being as we are. It is the being as we are within. That lightbody being within is connected with everything, the whole world, the whole universe, every universe, every time, every dimension, every mind, and every experience.

All of this knowledge is available to the master. The apprentice needs to limit their focus so that they do not clutter up their mind with everything. They must focus on their own studies. To be a lightbody worker means to eventually focus on a professional career in lightbody as a lightbody healer, scholar, physician, or in another discipline in lightbody work.

Using the lightbody is part of the consciousness sharing that goes beyond the regular world. By communicating by spirit and mind one may even know when adversaries or competitors are spying upon them. It is an advantage. Having these abilities, these lightbody skills, definitely helps in the real world.

The real world consists of people with lightbodies. How they use their lightbody skills can mean success or failure in the real world. To use the lightbody skills to see what is ahead is what lightbody is about too. To manifest one's aspirations in time is part of lightbody. Lightbody for some cultures means giving up and being poor and destitute, but it does not have to be that way. Lightbody empowers people to be successful.

The closer one is to who one is, the better one can be. If one has a real touch on one's skills and powers and learns how to use the lightbody energies, then one is on the way to success. One uses those skills in one's own world.

Lightbody training is not a substitute for regular education. It involves procedures that are common in all educational programs so there is nothing unique about this except the application of those principles to the lightbody world. Lightbody education should begin very young, in the womb, and through the formative years. As people become adults this knowledge should all be part of their relationships in their lightbody community. They will naturally know whom they are compatible with. Young people will not have to go through as much angst about dating. They will have a greater connection to their community, to those people that are available for dating, have similar vibrations, similar missions, and skills.

You can feel the world if you are in touch with your lightbody. You can feel other lightbodies in other people. You know instinctively who you are compatible with and can get along with. There is an interchange of energy that allows a possibility of love, friendship, comradeship, or just being associates, but in a good and friendly way. This allows people to naturally know who they like to hang out with. It is not just that a particular group of people gets together. Possibly they are together because they have a certain mind set. Many people have a certain vibe set.

That vibe set is an emanation of the lightbody. Lightbody emanations are part of the lightbody world. As people become more sensitive to their lightbody, they are able to harmonize more in their work environment, their school environment, and in the real world, because they feel the vibrations that people emit. They know how to make their energy waves work with the energy vibrations around them or else they bypass energy that they do not need to be around. Lightbody education allows people to be discerning about people who may not have the same harmonic or resonance. A lightbody worker cannot expect to harmonize with everybody. One can learn to harmonize with others who can be recognized by their particular frequency. One can emulate it and create a resonating frequency. It helps stimulate the apprentice to advance if they can resonate with their teacher.

The lightbody worker learns through experience. Activation of the lightbody abilities comes through education and the lightbody environment. As people in the lightbody community communicate and share experiences, they further their own lightbody education and the lightbody education of others. This entire process of lightbody sharing is part of what lightbody is about.

Why we have been suppressed in our lightbody knowledge for so long? That is a rather difficult subject. It takes patience. It takes discipline. It may take a religious background to effect lightbody changes.

When learning about lightbody and how to manifest lightbody, one has the challenge of not throwing one's lightbody around or bumping into places and annoying people. Beware of creating bad experiences for others and therefore for oneself possibly.

The student initially learns to be discerning about the extent of their lightbody and how it affects other people. That is why knowledge of the aura is important in lightbody education. The student learns how to use the lightbody in play, self-defense, and healing.

The manifestation of the lightbody by the lightbody master is a matter of using the skills that they have learned in the real world by creating portals of mind in space and time. These portals allow the individual master lightworker to travel to places where they accomplish the missions that they are assigned or choose.

The lightbody worker is part of a network of lightbody workers that exist throughout the universe and because of that they have certain privileges and certain abilities to travel to many different places. They share in the companionship of other lightbody masters.

One might wonder, where are these lightbody masters? They are everywhere. We just do not see them. If we are not calling for them and asking them to manifest, then they are probably doing other things, better things. Unless they can find a good reason for you to see them, then you might find a good reason for them to see you.

Lightbody education gives the student the ability to go to places of consciousness where they can learn to manifest their lightbody skills without being harmed or harming others. That is why a safe lightbody school is essential to master these skills and to cause no harm while you are learning them, because it is such a powerful experience. A lightbody school is a powerful place that it is difficult for people to take in without a through adjustment, preamble, and preparation.

Lightbody Mindset

The lightbody mindset is a consciousness, or a type of will, or a state of mind, that allows the lightbody user, the lightbody worker to manifest lightbody energy. The lightbody attitude is the setting up of one's consciousness to perform in the lightbody world, to use lightbody tools, to do lightbody deeds, and to perform lightbody miracles. Using lightbody tools is part of many cultural traditions. Although there are various procedures, the goal is usually to heal or enlighten. The lightbody actor and actress have a responsibility to know their talents and limitations as well. They have a certain set of talents that come with them, that are innate to them, because of who they are.

Every being has their own set of talents and their own set of lightbodies, but these bodies are limited by certain characteristics. Elephants have four legs and a trunk in their lightbody and birds have wings and feet in their lightbody.

Some animals have tails and horns in their lightbody. Even insects have lightbodies. They all have different forms and their lightbodies take those forms as well.

In most beings the lightbody exists within the physical body and does not leave the physical body until death. The lightbody is part and parcel of the physical body in most instances. The separation of the lightbody from the physical body is a matter of great concern and a matter of great danger as well.

The inexperienced apprentice who dares to take matters in his or hers own hands and uses lightbody as desired might find more than they want. Things might happen that go out of control. This is a basic danger in lightbody work.

There is definitely the sorcerer's apprentice problem. As one is learning lightbody, one has to be humble and know that impatience only causes trouble. One may not be ready to know everything now. One may need to learn a little later.

Lightspirit

Lightspirit is like the Holy Spirit except lightspirit is also energy. Lightbody is the manifestation of the lightspirit in a body, whereas lightspirit is like the Holy Spirit that is part of the Trinity: the Father, the Son, and the Holy Spirit. Most call this spirit the Blessed Spirit. The Blessed Spirit is the spirit that is most used in lightbody healing technology. Learning lightspirit and the use of lightspirit is part of lightbody technology.

Lightspirit is energy. It is termed spirit energy or spiritual energy. Spirit energy resides in many places. The highest or most beautiful is the Blessed Spirit or the Holy Spirit. As individual spirits, we have resonance with the Holy Spirit to certain degrees depending on our spirit energy, frequency, and attributes.

The manifestation of Holy Spirit by the physical body of the apprentice or lightbody master is done through the attendance of the Blessed Spirit. Other attending spirits may offer instruction and guidance in the manifestation of spirit energy, of lightspirit energy. Lightspirit energy is the energy used to perform healing miracles, psychic surgery, visionary portal openings, and reality portal openings to different dimensional realms.

Using lightspirit is essential in mastering lightbody technology. Lightspirit is a general term that deals with energy or energy field, but it is an actual stratum of reality. It is a vibration rate that is filled with a vibrating energy, which is like light energy.

Lightenergy may be independent of particularly directed spirit energy. The forces that can control lightspirit are the forces that are available to the lightbody. Lightbody manifestation of lightspirit is made possible through the disciplined practices of the master or apprentice. The lightspirit master must have mastery of the lightbody to use the lightbody as a conduit for the Holy Spirit in the work. To use lightspirit forces in the work involves bringing lightspirit energy to a point of focus. This is done through a focus of mentally directed energy. The individual apprentice or master creates a lightspirit portal for energy of this nature to be transmitted from a realm that is described as a stratum of being. It is from that realm, that stratum, that vibratory place, that this Holy Spirit energy is able to infiltrate our reality.

The lightspirit worker creates those portals. In use of the lightbody, the lightspirit worker is able to travel to different places out of the physical body to perform the spirit work.

The lightbody worker may become a lightbody surgeon. They can learn how to do psychic surgery. This involves going to realms that are other than normal by using portals to travel through these psychic spaces. These psychic portals may be opened at any time. Psychic portals can be moved to different places in the proximity where the innovator, imaginator, or manifester is able to project it. Learning to project these manifestations through lightbody consciousness is a matter of training.

This is either a skill or a second sense. These manifest energies or structures can emanate from the physical body and the lightbody and are used to perform various tasks.

By using your imagination as an entity in control of your lightbody, you can project that lightbody into action. These actions can influence a lightbody at another location, such as a lightbody patient who needs a certain operation. These procedures are well-known. Using the lightbody mind to do the initial diagnosis of a lightbody problem is part of the procedure.

One can be a lightbody in oneself, a lightbody anywhere, and a lightbody with a patient. It requires a certain amount of faith to transcend ordinary lightbody boundaries. To penetrate a physical being with one's physical hands is called psychic surgery. This is an attribute of some of the Philippine psychic surgeons.

To do other forms of psychic surgery is an ability that others might accomplish if they are truly skilled or devoted to becoming skilled in it. Becoming a multidimensional being is a challenge for anybody.

Spirit thought, or light thought is what connects the human being and their consciousness with the spirit. This is a communication that we would call light thinking or thinking in the light. It is a manifestation of consciousness that is in the flow of reality, of the light reality.

This means that the consciousness of the physical human being, the conscious mind driven by the body, is actually activating the mental-intellectual connectivity or it is being activated by it. The physical body can act as a channel for the intelligence or information of a spirit nature that we would call lightbody information, lightbody learning, lightbody thinking, and lightbody technology. Understanding this involves lightbody visualizations and exercises for the apprentice.

In understanding lightbody, one has to understand the implications of the physical body's connection to the lightbody and the lightspirit emanations from the lightbody. The lightspirit can be seen as emanations from the physical body, or from the lightbody if the lightbody is separated from the body. In looking at the lightbody spirit, the lightbody is in communication with the lightbody spirit energy.

The lightbody can direct the energy, which is Holy Spirit energy, from various parts of the body. If it were a human body, emanations of spirit energy could be from the hands, feet, head, mouth, or other parts of the body and especially the chakras. Lightbody communication with lightbody energy is a matter of manipulation of the lightbody spirit or spirit energy.

This is a universal energy that is manifest in the universe and available to lightbody masters and lightbody apprentices. Using this energy is a matter of practice and discipline. It takes practice to learn the use of lightbody energy, especially if the individual in their physical form wants to use their lightbody energy at any distance.

Otherwise, their lightbody may only be effective in working at short distances, in close contact, or in massage. Lightbody massage is based on using the lightbody to direct the human body in massage techniques. These therapies that the lightbody provides have additional power because they use lightbody energy. Lightbody energy is the basis of this whole energetic experience.

The lightbody energy that is transferred through lightbody massage is lightbody to lightbody, lightbody to human body, and lightbody to other bodies. The entire process of healing through lightbody is a multilevel or multilayer process. Each of these has its attributes that are classifiable by the functions and techniques that allow certain forms of healing to occur. The techniques are based on parts of the anatomy and other bodies such as the psychological, emotional, and spiritual bodies.

Lightbody can be used in this communicative healing. How close is the lightworker from the physical body that contains the lightbody? Are the lightworker's hands above the physical body? How far are the hands from the physical body? How many inches? How many feet? A world away?

Are the lightbody technician's physical hands actually penetrating the patient's physical body? Are the lighthands actually penetrating the physical body? All that has to be seen. The intelligence behind this phenomenon is lightbody intelligence. This is a combination of intelligence that is embodied in the hand of the lightbody technician and the technician's intelligence.

The lightbody technician usually uses their hands as the primary tool for lightbody work. Communication with the hand from the mind is essential. Proper communication between the hand and the mind is accomplished by performing lightbody synchronization of the mental factor with the physical factor.

Establishing the lightbody healing manifestation is a matter of establishing the presence of the lightbody formula. The formula might be a code or a sacred text such as the Bible. Other sacred texts or symbols can be used.

Using this lightbody intelligence in one's hands allows one to use greater intelligence than is possible by using pure spirit energy. Undirected spirit energy has a consequence of being undirected, so it is ineffective in some cases.

Lightbody illumination occurs when lightbody is able to transfer seed thoughts, or packets, or pods of information that are like little songs or little realizations that can be short or long, but they occupy a space in the mind.

These lightbody luminous illuminations are part of the lightbody transference of wisdom that occurs throughout space and time within entire lineages and peoples that grow together, those being families and spirits that occupy various forms such as plants, animals, and even rocks.

What is occurring when lightbody information is exchanged is that the lightbody people are actually lifting each other in this mutual support. Lightbody is something that helps everybody. By connecting and by being a light person, one can help other people achieve their goals too.

Those that emanate this spirit energy usually have a natural talent. The spirit energy should be good and possibly healing if it emanates at a good frequency. Communication with the spirit is essential in performing lightbody healing, lightbody surgery, lightbody psychic surgery, and illuminating surgeries.

Illuminating surgeries involve the illumination of the participant or the patient through the illumination of their own psychic intelligence channels or their own lightbody intelligences. These lightbody intelligences can achieve resonance with the lightbody master. In this case the resonance could be between the lightbody master and the lightbody apprentice.

To establish the lightbody intelligence factor, the lightbody master will establish a resonance within the lightbody apprentice. Through that resonance the master will activate either manuscript or symbol formulas within the apprentice's lightbody appendages. The master will instruct the apprentice in the operation of the lightbody technology.

The lightbody master is able to influence the apprentice in their advancement. This is done through lightbody directions, directives, instructions, and formulas to follow. These can be through performing various actions, rituals, prayers and exercises in conformity with their own religion or lightbody agenda. Lightbody training involves training across the spectrum. The training eventually focuses in on particular lightbody fields of endeavor.

These fields can be classified by their presence in the spiritual world or in the physical world. Lightbody intelligence can be transferred either partially or totally, depending on the transfer rate. This is similar to a bit rate. Information transfer can be total and immediate. The ability of the apprentice to comprehend the information may take a considerable time.

Lightbody uses of the spirit energy need training as well. The training can be installed in the apprentice through direct activation of the apprentice's lightbody energy and lightbody tools that are embedded in their lightbody hands and in their other lightbody tool appendages. The ability of the lightbody to use these tools may depend on the training and the experience of the apprentice.

This training has to be directed in a manner that accomplishes the greatest amount of training in the least amount of time. The amount of information is very great and the chance of making mistakes is even greater if the apprentice's efforts are not directed. If they are misdirected or undirected, there will be problems. If intelligence is not transferred properly it cannot be properly applied.

It is unfortunate that difficulties will arise in these situations if the apprentice is not fully aware of their responsibilities before starting. The teacher must have an unwavering support for the student's progress in these efforts. The consequences are such that improper training can lead to psychological, emotional, spiritual, and physical difficulties.

The use of lightbody technology is the use of lightbody spirit. Lightbody spirit is the spirit that one has and it is like the Holy Spirit. The Holy Spirit in its work as either material or non-material is within many comprehensional realms. If we can conceive of spirit in some form in our reality, then we can conceive of the world as something that can be enlightened by the presence of the spirit.

The spirit is enlightening. The spirit is light. As we have had the age of Our Father and the age of The Son, these times of the new millennium may be the time of the Holy Spirit and the dispensation of the Holy Spirit into humanity. In the understanding of this Holy Spirit, this age, and this dispensation from the Holy Spirit into this world, one can understand that the spirit is giving all spiritual energy to the world. Because of this, the vibration of the world is becoming more inundated by the energy of the Holy Spirit. The indication of people manifesting greater amounts of spiritual energy in their bodies is a manifestation of the greater availability of the spiritual energy and of the times we are in.

As the times change towards more influence of the Holy Spirit, the Holy Blessed Spirit will have more effect in the lives of everyone. This effect will be measured in the experiences and phenomena that can be attributed to the Holy Spirit. This means that supernatural phenomena will have a particular significance. Mysterious and unexplained phenomena will have to be examined in its relationship to the Holy Spirit.

The Holy Spirit is working in ways that will allow It to do things to change the world towards what It desires it to be, working in the ways that It does. Working in the ways that the Holy Spirit has, the Holy Spirit extends Its influence throughout the world, throughout each individual, throughout each spirit. It makes connection to each and every one.

The Age of the Holy Spirit has come. The new millennium has great potential to fulfill all the ideals of humanity, whatever they may be. The Holy Spirit is One that extends through all humanity no matter what their belief, no matter what faith they were born with, or converted to, or they will conform to. The Holy Spirit is universal and it is within us all. One can pray in any religion and still have the Holy Spirit.

The Holy Spirit is everywhere and the Holy Spirit has time to be with you. The Holy Spirit is filling all of you. The Holy Spirit is the influence of this new age. The Holy Spirit has a great message, a great duty, and great destiny for us all.

What we do and what we become in this new age depends on our connection to this Holy Spirit and all of our other beliefs. The Holy Spirit has connection to this time because of the intelligence of this time.

Lightbody Masters

Lightbody technology involves the use of lightbody in a way that is possible by using the lightbody methods and procedures that are learned from the lightbody masters. The lightbody masters have knowledge because they have learned that knowledge or acquired that knowledge by transference, implants or other means. The apprentice learns the knowledge by those means as well. The best way is through direct experience taught by the master.

The apprentice has many methods available for learning lightbody technology. In the practice of lightbody technology the apprentices do not have to learn everything, only what is necessary to achieve their own goals. Being aware of what they can do in total is good. It allows the individual apprentice to choose their path of lightbody fulfillment.

Using these abilities, energies, or lightbody powers involves the use of advanced imaginary abilities. This is normally gained through having a mindset that is based on an ability to construct images in the imagination or the mind's eye to do the lightbody work. This has often been called magic. The way this works is by working in the other world, the lightbody world. This is a world we all go to or in at times and all visit. Normally we have our own lightbody right within us all the time, or most of the time.

It is only on occasion that we travel out with our lightbody and those occasions are usually rare. It is normally only during sleep, accidents, or death that the lightbody leaves the physical body. The leaving of the physical body by the lightbody has to be a very guarded experience. It has to be taught.

The person practicing lightbody manipulation or magic has to know how to work their lightbody without letting their physical body undergo harm. The problem with lightbody technology is that it requires a certain amount of energy. That energy is normally so great that it depletes the physical body. It causes the physical body to age faster, to look older, and to be less functional if the healer or lightbody worker is not able to use that lightbody energy effectively.

The lightbody workers must look after themselves first before they even attempt some of this lightbody work. They know that they are in danger of being depleted of their lightbody energy. Lightbody energy is like any other energy. It is not something that one can give away without needing to have it replenished.

It is something that one can generate, transfer, and can make available either through the aura or through the lightbody. The lightbody world is a light-body world. It is a world where the lightbody can go and do its work and it has direct contact with the physical world.

Where you go with your lightbody is not always where you can go in your physical body. There are places that the physical body is not able to go that the lightbody can go to such as out in space, to different planets, or deep under the earth. Maybe our human technology will improve at some point.

To use lightbody enables the lightbody practitioner, or lightbody master, to do all sorts of things in their pursuit of their own fortune in this world. They must look after themselves first. This involves looking after their health, finances, fortune, career, status, and family.

Protecting oneself is all part of being a lightbody worker. To be part of the lightbody world is to have an inner connection that is supportive so there is not a loss, but a building together. This mutual support from all within the network of the lightbody workers enables the lightbody work to go on.

Although there are lightbodies in everyone and the lightbody worker can see that, the lightbody workers only work with their own patients or their own charges. These people are teaching their apprentices, students, and those they are working with in their families, or otherwise. Lightbody work can take many forms. Lightbody work is done by many religions. The work can occur in different times and spaces.

This work is something one might be doing now. One might be working on something in the future or working on something in the past. What is this work? It is a joining of all these things together that the lightbody is able to do. The lightbody worker has to know how to do that. That is why they follow different procedures to get different things done.

One has to do things in certain ways, with certain virtual parameters or templates, to accomplish the lightbody work. One can learn these kinds of things because they are basic and can be taught by a lightbody master in a lightbody school.

The lightbody apprentice needs to know exactly what they need to know. This means that they need to know that there are a set of goals and procedures that can be taught. One can teach oneself, but what if one tries to learn this by oneself without a teacher or a master? What if something goes wrong?

What if one opens up oneself the wrong way? Having a bad master might be as bad or worse. The lightbody worker has to beware and know what they are getting into and how they are getting into it. That is why having knowledge of the lightbody world is essential. To know where you are going and being in a place to know where you are coming from is also good. It lends to your whole experience in the here and now. By seeing in the lightbody world, you see where you are going to be and where you have been.

That means you can have a visual and auditory experience of lightbody life in previous lives, in future lives, in alternate lives, and other worlds. These are all available to the lightbody worker. The lightbody master has a tap in the universe, in their own lineage, in their own skills, and in their own identity. It is not lost. It is within your lightbody knowledge. It is within the lightbody identity. It is within your identity. What you learn is part of your

31

identity. What you do is part of your identity. What you regret is part of your identity. What you cherish is part of your identity.

Lineal remembrances are part of the heritage of all lineage members. Being a lineage member means you are entitled to all lineage privileges and those lineage privileges include the privilege to live, eat, and reproduce in the environment you are born in. There are many variations on the themes of life and lineage in the world. That is why getting along is important. That is why respecting lineages is important. That is why God has respected all lineages and has given all lineages the support of the Holy Spirit. The Holy Spirit works through the lineages and the religions all over the world.

There are many things that go into making the lightbody. What happens is that the lightbody has experiences that it can accumulate through time. Lightbody experience can be accessed by that individual lightbody or by other lightbodies.

The lightbody archive of knowledge is eternal. Accessing of the knowledge archives gives great strength to one's lightbody knowledge. This lightbody knowledge extends across the worlds and across the universe.

Where does one find such lightbody knowledge? In these cases it is found within the individual. It is found within you. It is found within your time, your space, and your mind. How does one do it? How is it accomplished?

It can be accomplished in various manners. The easiest manner is to follow a procedure that allows one to develop lightbody skills. Knowing about lightbody is the first thing. To manifest your lightbody out in the world is the second thing. That is why one learns lightbody manifestation skills. Lightbody communication skills are the next stage.

Those three steps are the first steps in lightbody. The first step in lightbody is realization of your lightbody. That means realization of you, of you and yourself, or you outside of yourself. That is why lightbody education is so important.

Where are you going to find the you that is outside yourself if it is not going to leave you? How do you leave you? How do you become part of something else, such as the greater whole? How do you extend? How is that extension possible? What does that mean? Why would one want to do that? How is that done if one wants to?

Those questions are answerable. Those things are part of lightbody knowledge. Those things are part of the experience that the master teaches the apprentice. That knowledge is part of the overall knowledgebase of lightbody wisdom. Lightbody wisdom extends through time and extends through space to other minds and alien minds. One can draw upon lightbody wisdom throughout space and time.

The application of lightbody wisdom is possible if the apprentice can use their innate skills to do the visualization exercises, the concentration exercises, the energy exercises, the devotional exercises, and the manifestation exercises as well.

There are many ways in which one learns how to manifest the lightbody energy, the lightbody being, and the lightbody. To be oneself outside oneself, to be oneself in another world, in another realm, takes quite an amount of concentration. That is why lightbody training is essential.

Lightbody concentration is necessary because you need to remember exactly what you are doing when you are doing it, why you are doing it, the exact procedures that you are going to use to do what you must do and want to do.

Getting lost in procedures can be very time-consuming. When the procedure is not followed it can mean difficulties, setbacks, and expensive kinds of problems. By being prepared, by having a foreknowledge of what one is going to do, by having back-up systems, and by having common sense, allows the lightbody worker to work in a way that can effect change throughout the worlds that they need to effect.

Lightbody Apprentice

Beginning the next phase in the apprentice's development depends on the timing of the apprentice's cycle of knowledge. This knowledge can be transmitted telepathically, orally, and to a certain extent written, as clues anyway. The master determines the full extent of the apprentice phase. The development that is available to the student is determined by the master's ability, time, and other factors.

The impact of the teaching upon the apprentice may cause changes in the apprentice. As the apprentice grows and knows more, he or she questions more and then knows less. One knows so much and knows that is so little. The big dilemma for the student is to know when to pursue a certain teaching from the master.

The knowledge gained by the student is only gained through trust in the teacher as being the conveyor of that knowledge. The teacher needs assurances of the disciple or apprentice's intentions. That can be determined by a certain cash obligation or property given for the exchange of the work, determined by the master and apprentice. The requirements of the master are usually fully determined by the master, or the masters, or directors, such as the board of directors.

The pursuit of these apprenticeship programs by the individual is with the knowledge that they have certain obligations to the teacher, and even to the school or the lineage that they belong or learn the practice from. That primarily means to hold the honor truly and to honorably be the apprentice of the master, and to carry on the lineage without deviating from it for one's own deviating purposes. This fully represents the high ideals of the lineage and the teaching. When the apprentice begins the program they know that the ideals that they are seeking are in harmony with their personal ideals. This makes the training so much easier and this teaching so much more understandable.

The pursuit of the knowledge allows individuals to transcend their normal conscious awareness and to become part of a greater awareness. The enthusiasm in which the apprentice or disciple pursues this will normally determine the speed in which they will achieve the results that they are trying to obtain.

In these pursuits as in the pursuits of other talents or modes of awareness, the individual needs to be aware of their own limitations. One hopes to transcend them in some way. That is part of this entire process. The individual's ability to be a disciple or apprentice will usually determine the height of what can be attained. With the master's blessings there may be more.

There is a law of give and return. That what one gives is what one gets. What you get is what you give. It becomes a great cycle of giving, growing, learning, and showing. By becoming what we are together, by sharing the knowledge that we have, by sharing the good knowledge, we can become better together.

In considering the weaknesses of the apprentice, the master might allow various regimes of routines or paths towards a certain level of awareness that can occur within a certain time frame. In the unfoldment of the psychic ability necessary to use the light-form, lightbeing, and lightbody in effective practice, the individual aspiring to these abilities must have dedication to these principles.

The principles laid out are those of non-harm and non-greed. This means taking only for oneself, and to respect the privacy of others and their own environment. In general, do not hassle people. Try to start by being good when you are out there, performing your exercises. Strive to attain the purposes you set yourself to do in your lightbody work.

The agreement that you make in the lightbody work will give you a matter of freedom to accomplish the work without great oversight if you are working with your full imagination and willpower. If you are intuitive and listening, your guides should provide wisdom that guides in the unfoldment of your abilities, psychic or otherwise.

The entire full spectrum of a person's ability is necessary in this work. Individuals intending to do this work cannot shy off from their pursuit of normal life, jobs, obligations, relationships, and everything else that goes with reality. These lightbody experiences are supplemental. The farther one is from the lightbody realm the less the person is able to experience the total of reality.

In this pursuit the individual feels the greater whole. By becoming part of the greater whole and by expanding beyond themselves, they become more than who they are and can share that with others. This pursuit is joyous because it allows people to share more, be more, and to become more, as they pursue their own desires and pleasures together.

Play is the first step in the pursuit of lightbody wisdom. Play begins as the parents play with the child in ways that are giving and loving. People can play in childish ways and play in ways that expand their abilities in ways that they may not know at first. They will feel their abilities expand as they move their lightbody from themselves outward and are then able to place it at different locations. This is sometimes known as bi-location. This is a consequence or an attribute of lightbody because lightbody can become a bi-located entity that is directed by consciousness. You can bi-locate by having your physical body in a somnolent state or in deep meditation.

Lightbodies associated with an individual may be single or multiple. The fracturing of lightbodies and their frequency responses are not as responsible if they are multiple, and therefore lightbody singularity is preferred.

The lightbody experience is one in which individuals can benefit from being together because they can share the resonance of lightbody. Lightbody resonance is equal to harmonizing at a particular frequency of lightbody. That can become a starting point for cooperation and lightbody play. Lightbody play involves multiple lightbodies in proximity, usually within a foot or closer, and often touching and merging, along with other lightbody exercises.

These exercises can be termed play although they can become difficult. The lightbody exercises that will be presented are presented as games. The exercise and its intensity are up to those playing these lightbody games. Lightbody games are intended to enhance the player's ability. They enhance the player's ability to use their lightbody in space and time.

It is best if the people playing lightbody are within the same room when they learn to play, approximately within ten feet to each other. That distance can grow to be across the room or much greater distances, and then at much greater distances such as across the country, and so forth. The first exercises in this may involve using the lightbody in exercises in a room of about thirty feet by fifteen feet or bigger. This is a good area for about ten people.

The lightbody experience is not one that one will easily forget because it is so really strange. It could be forgotten if you are only able to experience it in a state of consciousness that is foreign from your own. Do not go there unless you are ready to experience your lightbody energy. It is not easy to experience lightbody energy without going to a place where you can use your lightbody. That place is not easily attained.

The lightbody experience becomes more enhanced in the presence of people that are pursuing lightbody experience and lightbody intelligence. This involves knowing how to use the lightbody in relation to the physical body. In early training it is best to show the individual apprentice how to use the physical body in lightbody exercises so they have an idea of what to do.

The lightbody is a projection of the physical body and mind although it can take other forms. Lightbody projections from the self and consciousness into the world and into other dimensions, space and time, and other places, are normally done for investigation, re-living, adventure, and spiritual purposes. Recreational purposes are the real draw to the lightbody experience. Many want the pleasures of lightlove, lightbody sex and joy.

Lightbody is something that many people experience and have experience with because it is part of our human ability to have lightbody. It is just that we are not always aware of that lightbody. That lightbody is usually within you. You have your own lightbody within you and I have my lightbody within me.

In our normal life one has a lightbody within. Sometimes the lightbody may be jolted from the body if one is in an accident or hurt. One's physical eyes might be looking up while one's lightbody is above looking down. As the lightbody leaves the physical body it sometimes leaves an impression on this world too. There are many vibrations that can occur when the lightbody is affected because the lightbody is part of one's body. It is often associated with the aura, but it is not the aura.

Lightbody beings are like spirits. They are connected with the body of the living being with an intelligence that has direction, hopefully. If the lightbody is misdirected, devious forces may be directing it. That must be avoided. There has to be caution when playing with lightbody.

Lightbody is something that people can normally learn without much training. The more training one has the better one is able to cope with the abilities that develop from using those abilities.

Lightbody play is a form of developing one's abilities in lightbody. Lightbody play means doing these exercises with certain degrees of proficiency along the way. Most of these exercises are repetitive in nature or have various repetitive formats. One can do various color changes to one's lightbody. Take your lightbody through the spectrum of the rainbow. That might be an exercise that you excel in.

One might be called to do a patterning of one's lightbody in other lightbody exercises. Other interesting challenges await the apprentice during lightbody training. Knowing what to do with lightbody is a matter of training as well. Being effective with your lightbody is the whole reason of learning with your lightbody.

The principles of lightbody are usually guided by morals and by cultural or religious perceptions of lightbody. Lightbody is not limited to any particular religion or intelligence group. Lightbody is something that has been seen around the world for ages and called different things.

In using lightbody or being one with one's lightbody, one is relying on knowledge of traditions that extend back through time. Lightbody knowledge extends back through cultures and lineages that have great experience with lightbody. Lightbody in itself is a study that allows people to become more than themselves because they can order the universe around them through their own lightbody emanations.

Lightbodies are such that they are able to operate in ways that human bodies sometimes cannot. They can establish vibrations in the space and time realm where the human cannot. They can be intelligent advisors, observers, movers and shakers in realms that the human may not be able to attend to.

The lightbody is an extension of oneself. How does it operate in the world? Some cultures have called the lightworker a shaman, witch, or wizard. Various names throughout the world were given to these individuals that were able to manifest themselves through their lightbodies and had special abilities. Those abilities are documented, sometimes believable and sometimes not. Exaggerated claims are extremely easy to make. Take any of this lightbody knowledge and training with a grain of salt. What may be true for me may not be true for you. It may not even work for me in the way that it could work for someone that was better trained than myself.

Part of the knowledge of lightbody is given to certain individuals and part of it is earned through the efforts of other individuals. It is all an ongoing effort. It is a group effort of all individuals involved in lightbody study and the lightbody experience around the world.

Why are so many people involved in it? Because of the benefits to humanity that are possible through lightbody participation and lightbody extension. Lightbody is a way of healing which is seen in the lightbody workers in the Philippines using faith healing. Lightbody has many great traditions.

Having control of one's lightbody is part of being a real spiritual person or a real religious person. In many cases, having faith in the miracles that most religions attest to is having faith in lightbody.

If one needs to gather intelligence through the world, lightbody training can become a form of intelligence gathering. Training through teachers, classes, or telepathically leads the individual aspirant or apprentice to greater knowledge. The knowledge pursued is an appetizer.

The wisdom gained is so much greater than just knowledge, words, or science because it is a wisdom that extends through space and time. One type of wisdom might be knowledge of how the universe works in waves. If the individual could feel the waves, they would be in tune with that knowledge.

That knowledge extends beyond equations or other forms of logic. The intuitive ability of the person pursuing this knowledge should be as great as their desire to know it. They should have no problem grasping concepts beyond their normal understanding.

These abilities are not gained. They are intuitive. The individual can pick them up through vibrations going on in their class, from their teachers, from their lineage, or in their world. It is all around. It is available to the individual who is able to tune into their desired topic and desired frequency of destiny.

The whole frequency of life is preserved within a space-time matrix of awareness that extends through space and time. It is available to the archivist, aspirant, and apprentice who can browse through it. The masters use this matrix of awareness to great advantage for their own purposes. It is good for all.

The apprentice can use their abilities to a certain degree. The master limits the student's permission to accomplish certain things, such as being a teacher before they are ready or sharing information that cannot be shared. This is to protect the student, school, and master.

The entire structure of trust is built upon a relationship that the student, apprentice, aspirant, or disciple builds with their college, school, church, seminary, monastery, or retreat. This allows the individual to pursue a format that is available to many, but follows a certain procedure or guideline that makes it palatable. This is within the scope of the people that need to participate, or want to participate, or can participate.

The necessity of doing these things with finesse and the need to do these things with knowledge of the individual apprentice's desires is paramount. That requires a pre-enlightenment training agreement that gives the school a clear idea of the intentions of the aspirant so that there are no questions later, or fewer questions later.

The aspirant or apprentice's obligations to the school extend from the moment they agree because of the extreme availability of the knowledge that they will pursue. It is usually to the school and apprentice's advantage that the financial obligations are fulfilled first. That way they do not feel any guilt about the payment. The lightbody activation may happen very suddenly or it may take months. It may take a year. It depends on the apprentice's time and ability.

It may take years for certain individuals to pursue and get to their level. They may have to accept this because of limited time, resources or ability. Those things are understandable and someone might say, "It took me years to get through school, and it took me a few more years to get through the psychic training for my lightbody."

The lightbody exercises allow individuals to go at their own pace. Once the students see how easy the exercises are, and what their formats are, they can actually gain their skills in a much shorter time if they are able to play along. They can gain a greater magnitude of skill, knowledge, and ability to perform the things that they wish to do with their lightbody.

Lightbody is a general topic. It does not lend itself to any particular thing except as the individual is inclined to apply it. The individual is left to pursue their own will in lightbody technology, yet they must follow the principles and laws of physics and faith.

If they pursue their own destiny they might be helped along by the general rhythm of reality and the flows of destiny. If they are swept up in those currents they may find themselves in places and times that give them greater insight, power, and ability to fulfill their own destiny.

This is the greatness that is available to those who pursue this training. The apprentice has an ability to succeed where others may not dare to try. This ability gives the apprentice an ability to look further, to be more intelligent, to have a greater ability to concentrate, to have an intelligent plan, and to develop the foresight to carry it out intelligently as well.

There are many challenges and these are just a few. The actual results are something that we sometimes may not appreciate. They may not have the effect that we want, or we may not see the effect, or the effect may not be known for some time.

It is not always easy to judge the effect of lightbody technology upon reality until you are able to effect the ability within yourself and to actually manipulate reality with some intensity. That is why training and light ability is what is necessary.

Light ability is something that allows the person to be especially capable of preserving themselves in their own physical body. They are able to keep their physical body alive when they are using their lightbody in other pursuits. This involves split intelligence and a monitoring that goes beyond right-left brain. This is real concentration and it is not something easily attained. This split intelligence can be attained through great concentration.

Once it is attained, the concentration is not necessary. It is an ability. It is like riding a bike or driving a car or anything else. You just learn it and it is there. The light ability that a person enjoys is the ability to project themselves beyond themselves and then do more. They have more to do and they can do more because they are more.

The projection of oneself into the lightbody is usually by being more than you are and by having your lightbody as yourself. This means separating your lightbody from your physical body and seeing your lightbody in front of you. Project your experience into that lightbody. Take that lightbody. See that lightbody. Move that lightbody through your projection of will. Experience a connection to that lightbody. If you do not have a connection, it may not be your lightbody. Say goodbye if it bothers you.

Lightbody experience is such that you recognize you because you are you and you recognize other beings because they are they. You recognize your connection to your lightbody through your psychic cord, through your umbilical cord at the navel, normally. Sometimes there are other connections such as in the heart and in the third eye and other connections that extend through space and time. Connecting the lightbody through those methodologies allows the individual to go to great extents and to places in space and time and access knowledge that is not available through normal consciousness.

These lightbody excursions may cause a great snap back when the individual's consciousness returns to the physical body. The lightbody has traveled through great amounts of space and time and returned to the physical body. The physical body is not lonely without its lightbody. The lightbody should only be gone for as long as it can maintain its lightform with the concentration of the physical body.

A lightbody usually does not want to leave the physical body behind. It cannot retain its own concentration on being separate from its own physical being for too long. The physical body needs to maintain its physical realities and rhythms, its ability to breath and its functions. The lightbody being has to be responsible for the physical being when it is the intelligent one.

Projecting one's being and intelligence through space and time is quite a stretch of thought. Taking one's individuality and sharing oneself through space and time allows one to feel much more and much further than one normally could. During excursions into those other realms, one has separation from the physical body and that separation can sometimes be dangerous.

Those using lightbody technology must learn about the problems that arise from using the lightbody. The dangers of lightbody technology include dangers to the physical self, the mental self, spiritual self, the psychological self, the emotional self, and the auric self. All of these selves get shaken up when one starts using lightbody technology.

Being a lightbody person or a person that can use lightbody means that one is doing things that are out of the ordinary. One might cause trouble to the normal world and the normal body and bring on energies, illness, or even cure illnesses.

One cannot be sure what is going to happen until one starts doing lightbody. One wants to have the training of a teacher so one does not go too far with what one is not supposed to do. Not only that. One needs to know where one is going to go anyway.

Not having a teacher causes pain to the student and eventually the teacher has to retrain the student. That is a pain too.

Lightbody training and tutoring is something that some people are easy at giving, but it is something that should not be pursued without the right intentions. There are problems that can be incurred during lightbody training. If a teacher does not know how to accept the karmic obligations of training, then the individual student could be lost in limbo and only gain certain psychic abilities that cause them great damage, harm, and pain.

This is because greater awareness and sensibility may cause emotional stress. If the teacher is not there to help them for the rest of their life, they are stuck. A little may be too much for some people. They need so much more. It is like showing somebody how to feel, and then they cannot stop feeling ever again.

It is a double-edged sword one might say. It is a difficult task to pursue being a teacher of this knowledge. The impact it has is not only on the student, but also on the teacher. The eventual obligations and responsibilities go beyond the initial agreement. Something is going to occur, some training, some exercise, and some play. All of these things just lead deeper and deeper.

It is part of the whole process of using the lightbody. As people are becoming more accustomed to lightbody play, they are less inclined to be obsessive. They are more inclined to just have fun. It is like any other game except for the reasons that one plays it. A little bit more imagination is used because one is trying to do something miraculous, something that expands one's abilities beyond their abilities, something that gives one a reason to be greater than oneself.

The lightbody is something that most people intuitively feel. In hostile environments one must beware. Is their lightbody under attack by cruel stares from unsympathetic people? In a protected, safe environment one should be able to cooperate with others that are experiencing lightbody training and lightbody joy.

The lightbody community is a community of individual spirits that are united in space and time. An apprentice and a master can identify members of the lightbody community by sensing them with their lightbody senses.

The lightbody community not only exists on this earth, but it exists in other places in space and time. The apprentice might communicate with other lightbody intelligences in other spaces and times with the guidance of the master. In time, the apprentice may do this communication alone and learn from other lightbody masters in other parts of the universe.

The lightbody apprentice has available, upon agreeing to the terms of apprenticeship, the ability to learn ways to accelerate their lightbody consciousness that are almost unimaginable. The ability of the apprentice has to be expanded exponentially by doing feats of consciousness that are not normally available through normal conscious pathways and normal states of mind.

To achieve this state of consciousness, the apprentice must agree to a degree of psychic surgery or lightbody surgery. This allows blocks to be removed, the mind to be prepared, databases to be installed, and the connectivity in the universe to be manifested. This is a matter of fine-tuning. It is an adjustment of the apprentice and it is a matter of freewill. In many cultures it is rote and just a matter of how one grows up. That is what happens.

The lightbeing and lightbody technology can be transferred in manners that are both near and far. They can be transmitted across great distances using various technologies. There are limitations to the manifestation of lightbody beings in alternate realities. Lightbody instruments, vehicles, technologies, devices, and portals are all tools used by lightbody masters and apprentices.

Lightbody interchange is something that brings joy if done in the right manners under particular conditions. This means following the rules and regulations of lightbody play, lightbody love, and lightbody sex. All of these are part of the lightbody exercises that are part of the lightbody tradition. It is a tradition of family, love, and respect.

The lightbody is something that is a part of you, part of your family, tradition, lineage, culture, and religion, whatever that might be. It is just a factor of life. The lightbody emanates from the body and it is the body that essentially goes out and is able to enliven itself.

The lightbody information that the apprentice or master receives does not have to be from a source nearby. It can be from a source at a great distance. The information sources may need to hide how they install their information. They may give hints or clues about the information they are going to present.

A major example of this technology is the opening of space-time portals using crop circles. The appearance of various crop circles in various locations indicates the presence of beings that can project geometrical shapes onto multi-dimensional planes. The implication is that the mind concentrating on these structures of patterns can gain an ability. This ability is attained by concentrating on the geometrical form of the crop circle.

The format is a portal. Using the crop circle technology, which is a shape-based technology, the lightbeing and/or the lightbody user can use their mind to use a shape in a crop circle to manifest various degrees of consciousness. This opens portals to space-time and that allows communication with the beings that establish the crop circles. This meditation involves creating the two dimensional crop circle form in the mind's eye and then expanding it into a third dimension. Expand it to give it a form of three-dimensionality. Rotate it clockwise, counterclockwise, up, and down to see the different angles. Zoom in and zoom out.

Take the shape of the pattern and rotate it on its axis at various degrees, speeds, and directions. Contact the frequency and modulation of the rotating three-dimensional structure. The motion introduces the dimension of time. Unfold the inner patterns. Reverse the rotation of the circle and repeat the process.

Pictures may be seen through the vortex openings. As the vortex opens it may be accompanied by changes in frequency. There may be light emanations in the region surrounding the crop circle structure.

Using the lightbody technology, go into the portal or remain outside the portal and communicate from the portal's edge. See what it is, who it is, why it is, when it is, and where it is. These are all good journalistic questions.

The crop circles are knowledge transmission devices or tools. These are known as portals all over the world. There are various portals of this nature. They are often found at temples. Temple sites have mystical implications that give rise to the building of temples in places where people can feel the presence of space-time portals.

These space-time portals are established through the mind and through concentration. Using these structures in consciousness to create the necessary space-time disturbance or shockwave establishes the portal. Lightbody technology is the technology that leads to the ability to have certain types of manifestation. It enables manifestation of auric shockwaves.

What that means is that the physical individual has to attain and maintain a harmony with their lightbeing. Their consciousness is connected with their lightbeing and they are able to manifest a shockwave on lightwave frequencies. These shockwaves are forces or forcewaves that emanate in physical types or ways that we can measure either theoretically, virtually, or physically when the equipment is available.

The energy manifestation that the lightbody worker creates through these shockwave emanations comes from their hands or from their body. It comes from particular places either on or in their body, outside their body, either on their aura or outside their aura. Within certain parameters, there may be manifestations of heat and tingling on the body of the participant's sensors, which may be their hands. There are manifestations of other forces, either healing or otherwise using shockwave emanation.

Lightbody emanations may appear at different places in space and time depending on the will of the activator of the lightbody, who is usually the person within the physical body. It is usually by invitation that people's lightbodies are allowed to participate in educational adventures and other visionary experiences. Lightbody phenomena may be experienced as visions of people, entities, places, other times, objects, or animals.

Maintaining portal boundaries is important and it takes a special structuring. To maintain a structure through space and time while activating one's mind in other dimensions takes exacting patience, skills, and discipline. The practitioner of lightbody work must do all these things simultaneously while maintaining their focus on the purpose and goal of their mission.

The use of prayer in establishing space-time portals is especially effective. As people are able to use their prayer, their minds directed in prayer, and their emotions directed in prayer, they are able to open up these space-time portals.

Techniques of Enlightenment

The psychic surgical methodology can be applied to techniques of enlightenment. The master or teacher will train the student in methods of helping others to attain their enlightenment as well. In these procedures the student is actually learning to become the teacher. It is a process that is eternal and a part of the entire teaching and learning process.

The student has to remember everything so they can reverse engineer their training as they train others when becoming the master teacher. The apprentice is in a position to improve upon methods, to document methods, and take various procedures into different directions.

There is much opportunity for the apprentice to investigate different ways in which they are going to become masters in the skill sets they are going to pursue. In the procedure towards learning to become a master, the apprentice will go through a series of mental or intellectual challenges based on the learning curve of the student or apprentice.

These challenges present the student with a set of problems, which must be solved. The set of problems are particular to the training they are in. The teacher needs to take them through the set without much distraction. This is not an easy task to do online because it requires concentration and guidance by the teacher in these methods.

Knowing the student is part of the teacher's responsibility. Learning about the student is one of the first things the master needs to do when encountering and accepting the student in this process. The master will have an ongoing relationship with the student that will develop from the moment they begin. It may begin before that through other contacts.

The intention of the relationship is most important as it starts. The intention to fulfill a particular goal or mission is the first part of undertaking one of the exercises. Some of the initial exercises of the psychic surgeon have nothing to do with surgery or the body and are more of a form of learning or education. This has to occur in any discipline in order that the apprentice learns what needs to be done to accomplish what they want to accomplish.

The teacher and the apprentice must agree on a schedule that allows this progress to occur. The apprentice's knowledgebase needs to be increased if the apprentice is going to become a master in a limited amount of time. This usually has to be condensed because of other reasons. The apprentice, teacher, and master would have to make plans for an intensive training.

Retreats are ideal situations for an orderly unfoldment of ability. The knowledgebase that the student needs to obtain can be obtained partially through books, explanations, and descriptions of the entire process, such as this. The entire teaching is done in a real world way.

The intelligence or the information has to be passed on in a manner that is most easily called telepathic or passed on through lineage. It is information that the user does not have to know. The process of enlightening the student or apprentice can occur over a certain amount of time so that the student is able to digest or understand what is occurring.

The training levels that are available to the apprentice depend upon their base point of knowledge, understanding, and ability. If they have a base of knowledge of the subject along with alternate experiences that give them insights, then they may be far on their way to being a more advanced student.

As with any learning experience, this requires patience, perseverance, and faith. There will be an unfoldment of knowledge that is going to be available to the student as time unfolds. The student needs to be patient. Being an apprentice means realizing that one is going to learn when one is ready to learn. It is not always easy to adjust oneself to higher learning or have the teacher make the time to do this work with and for one.

Understanding is an unfoldment that takes time. The unfoldment of particular concepts and procedures take explanations. Doing this with a student takes time. These procedures must be explained in a meaningful way that is understandable and teachable by the student.

The knowledge that the student is entitled to learn depends on the relationship the student has with the master or the teacher. It is usually based on a monetary arrangement or a more family oriented arrangement based on tradition. In any case, the obligations of the student and the teacher are profound and their obligations to each other are great.

In the unfoldment of the student's abilities, the student has to prepare their mind for a body of knowledge that surpasses their present body of knowledge. This body of knowledge may not in any way be understandable at first, or even perceptible. The problem that the student may have is that it is vague, obscure, and does not seem to have much cohesiveness at first. This is because the student may not have had the actual training in the knowledge yet. Having the knowledge and having the training in the knowledge, or actually "groking" the knowledge as the Heinlein book said, are different kinds of concepts.

The understanding of these procedures is part of a legacy and part of a tradition that allows the student to use this knowledge in their life and to pass this knowledge on as intended. This knowledge is a shared knowledge. It is shared between people and between spirits throughout time. This knowledge extends beyond our own world. It is knowledge of life, existence, and being.

The student should be curious about how to unfold other talents that the teacher may not have time available to teach. If they are in pursuit of a particular healing skill or knowledge set, they might venture out and find that information themselves. In most cases, because of our experience as individuals, we may be masters at one thing or another, but we cannot be masters of it all.

Until there is another conference of masters of healing, there can be no real agreement and no broad perspective of this entire field of study. In ancient times the best scholars in the Vedic world gathered in the writing of medical books and setting up schools of healing. Indeed, that needs to happen again. The practice of various ancient forms of lightbody healing must be returned to. The true arts have been neglected, forgotten, or lost.

Lost is probably the problem here because the literature is not especially full of instances of this technology. It may be possible that it was isolated and lost in a particular stratum of space-time. The uncovering of knowledge in this database and this stratabase has an implication for the furthering of knowledge in our time. The transmission of knowledge can occur over the centuries and over thousands of years. This is possible and is being demonstrated here.

The connection to learn from others is the connection of the teacher and the master and the apprentice or the student. These relationships allow the student to access a teaching database that extends through time. As the student learns these other techniques they are able to extend themselves through space and time. Their consciousness becomes part of the continuum. They have knowledge ready at all times depending upon the connections, associations, and alliances they make for the knowledge they are in pursuit of.

The framework of knowledge is already built. It has existed for thousands or perhaps of millions of years. It is only our understanding of this database of knowledge that gives us the ability to use it in our own existence, which is our human existence.

In our existence as humans we have the ability to use our body to generate forces; light forces from our body, from our auric emanations, from the aura, and the energy body produced by the living body and associated with the living body. It is possible to establish the energy fields or the energy portals necessary to create the healing environment that makes possible the faith of miraculous healings.

The training of the apprentice involves the training of the apprentice's body, mind, emotions, spirit, and soul. It is an entire process for the apprentice because they are entirely immersed in the experience of becoming a lightbody being. Associating their lightbody being with their physical being is a challenge.

Taking the time to be lightbody aware means that the person cares about their influence in the spirit realm as well as their physical presence. Given that, they do have certain obligations to be nice bodies, nice spirit bodies, and nice lightbodies. They are obligated not to cause mischief out there and to be careful. It is a big world.

The lightworld is one in which people have abilities that one does not have in this world. Learning to be a lightbody person or lightbody active means that one has to be physically active in this body, in this world, in this space in time. That is why the attention to the physical body is necessary for the apprentice. The apprentice's challenge is to be physically fit, mentally aware, and emotionally balanced. Having one's spirit focused in the higher realms means the student is ready for this lightbody training and apprenticeship.

The lightbody apprentice has many challenges, but the rewards are great. The rewards are taken in order. The lightbody aspirant or student has to accept that they are going through stages and not to expect more than they may be ready for, or more than they have time for.

The inspiration or knowledge enlightenment available at these different levels is dependant on the individual aspirants' or the apprentices' ability to pass tests at different levels. These tests are already set up. The teacher may inform the student about the tests and even show them how to take the test. Eventually the test is given and the student is observed taking the test.

The methods of taking the test are known and taught. Taking the test has to be observed. Certificates of accomplishment are awarded. The acknowledgement of the accomplishments of the student is necessary. Then they know and can do exactly what they are able to do within the wider scope of their mission.

What that implies is that the knowledge set is so vast that they need, as in any other school or educational situation, to have the particular day and talent that they are learning catalogued in a calendar. Their knowledge is set in a database. That has to be reviewable by themselves and those they are going to show and demonstrate their skills to. It should be possible for the apprentice to learn and memorize these skills and skill sets. When they become teachers they can pass them on, knowing exactly what is necessary in that set of skills and procedures.

The use of these psychic abilities to train, learn, and communicate is all part of the psychic experience. These abilities are necessary for being a psychic surgeon or a manipulator of space-time. Those who dare to learn this knowledge might share it. Having to know everything about these subjects is not easy. It is not an endeavor or study that you can take up and leave. It is with you through time.

What you learn you will retain and can call upon it at other times in space and in mind. Taking your time to learn and patiently discern the truth, the fact from the fantasy, is all worthwhile. It allows the individual to go to greater heights, knowing what is real, and knowing what might not be.

Taking steps to know what can happen is the purpose of the training. The training allows the individual to see how far they might go under the supervision and guidance of those who have gone before. They might know that such an adventure is risky. They do not know how far they can see with the proper training. Being such a great adventure, those who dare might wish to know that it is all worth the time and effort, especially if one is devoted to it.

55

Psychic surgery or other forms of lightbody healing are only part of the total picture. There are other aspects that can be considered as modules as well, such as psychic play, lightbody love, and lightbody sex. There is lightbody parenting, lightbody healing, which includes psychic surgery, the medical aspects of the psychic, and lightbody enlightenment.

Lightbody enlightenment is one of the modules that take a direct contact with the teacher through contact in the classroom or telepathically. These masters have an ability to transmit information either orally, through written manner, telepathically, or by knowledge implant. This is instant knowledge database transfer into the individual apprentice. If the manner in which the individual attains their information is through database duplication and implant, then it usually needs to be decompressed.

The decompression methodology varies between the different schools using their own databases. The decompression of spiritual experience helps the teachers or masters to help the apprentices or students. The decompression of experience, which is usually a visionary experience or dream experience, can reveal the extent to which the student is allowed to learn, and their level of learning.

The difference between consciousness in the learning level and normal consciousness may be very great. It is advisable that the apprentice establishes these different plateaus of consciousness with ease, to be able to find the higher realms with ease, and to shift into normal consciousness when necessary. The consciousness work is done on the lightbody levels.

The division of activities in the lightbody work includes the introductory work, which involves setting up the different parameters around the lightbody environment. In energizing the lightbody environment, include any individuals within the environment, the teacher or the master, and angels or the entities that are participating in the lightbody environment. The new environment may have various attributes such as a conference room or temple. The lightbody environment has limitations. These limitations are established by the security in the environment.

The lightbody environment is secured by various means. Lightbody force energy and psychic protection are described elsewhere. Lightbody activation of the individuals within the parameter of the lightbody circle being protected allows a focused activation of the individuals for the process. The process of instant enlightenment can occur through data based transmission, decompression, and eventual activation.

The database is usually installed through psychic means, implantation, training, and absorption. These methodologies are not exclusive. The transference of database information to the consciousness of the apprentice is based on the apprentice's time and ability to understand.

There may be knowledge within the apprentice that cannot be unlocked until the apprentice attains certain heights of consciousness. Those heights of consciousness unlock different plateaus of understanding and enlightenment that are pending in the advancement of the apprentice's training.

The enlightenment plateaus are visible by means of travel with the teacher or master. The apprentice can observe the different levels that they may attain through their own efforts. If they are lucky enough to have a teacher that allows safe lightbeing travel, lightbeing existence, and security in the lightbeing realm, they can observe what they have yet to attain.

Lightbody is a form of being, a form of existence, and a state of mind. The connectivity between lightbody, real body, and real mind is especially important and cannot be discounted. Deviations from the mission or breaking of lightbody consciousness can cause difficulties such as shock to the body or to the mind, loss of memory, loss of consciousness, or loss of life.

The consequence of misusing lightbody energy must be avoided because of extreme shock. Sensitive individuals are aware of the ebb and flow of energy within the space-time continuum. Those who are masters of the energy can feel the force and feel the energy. They can feel disturbances in the force and energy around them. Their lightbody is their antenna body and it allows them to feel the forces in the world at a distance. Their auric body is directly connected to their physical body, their mental body, and their senses.

In understanding lightbody it is necessary to understand the aura body and the chakra system. This is basically a form of technology based on the human body. The human body in its own particular design has design factors or capabilities that allow it to operate in the lightbody realm. This multiple capability is attributed to genetics or to God. These abilities are so great that just understanding them in their potential can cause an individual to have an enlightening experience.

Lightbody awareness and lightbody manifestation is all part of being a body in this physical world. There are few who can manipulate their own consciousness to go out and be more than who they are just in their body. Naturally, one's lightbody resides in their physical body except possibly for instances such as dreaming. The lightbody could then escape or go to other places in the normal routine of dreaming, traveling on those dream levels; those dream realms, or those lightbody realms.

Lightbody travelers are not totally protected by their own innocence. They are vulnerable to forces as they venture out of their physical bodies. Most people need to protect themselves by staying within their physical bodies. That means their lightbodies must maintain presence within their physical bodies and not venture out of them. Most people should not let their lightbody venture too far out of their auric field.

The lightbody may extend out from the body if it is energized. That can be done through the direction of the consciousness in the lightbody and through the willpower of the apprentice or master. This may be seen in the aura. The lightbody is a form of auric energy. It is able to go off and out from the physical body. The physical body does not limit the lightbody.

The lightbody is an experience of the physical body, of the consciousness of the activator, of the owner of the lightbody, and should not be manipulated by other bodies. That could occur if the owner of the lightbody is not careful. The more sensitive a person is to lightbody, the more able they are to see when others manipulate them. Those others may have power in the lightbody realm. Being lightbody sensitive, lightbody manipulators also have the ability to change energy fields around them. The energy fields in their inner relationships can be changed through light-body manipulation.

These energy changes occur in group situations, personal situations, encounter situations in daily life, on the street, in a restaurant, at work, and in other situations. The use of the lightbody is a universal fact. People have these abilities to extend themselves in circumstances where they live and how they live.

It is through the lightbody training that the person learns to use the lightbody in a way that furthers them. It is an ethically based training and can ultimately lead the person to a greater understanding, enlightenment, and closeness with God.

The eventual religious factors involved in lightbody training are inevitable. The nature of lightbody training allows the individual not only to fulfill their own desires, but it allows God to work within them to fulfill God's desires. The greater the individual becomes in their successes, the greater God is able to influence the individual and influence the world. Greater good is brought to the world through the influence and actions of the individual.

The lightbody training is an eternal training. It is a training that started many ages ago and will continue on for many ages. It is not a training that is limited to humans. It is a training practiced throughout this galaxy. It is a natural training or experience that conscious beings across the galaxy and across the universe have devised for their own use in relating to reality.

Reality includes lightbody reality. For instance, we all have seen or heard of angels and other lightbody beings. We are well-prepared by our religions, mythology, and legends. Lightbody exists. We know that although we may not be able to prove it.

Science may not have all the facts about lightbody. Religion has many experienced people that have seen lightbody, experienced lightbody, have great religious belief in these lightbody beings existence, and faith that these lightbody experiences did occur. These are the miracles and other lightbody manifestations seen as visions at Fatima and other places. These lightbeings are able to manifest themselves in visions, in minds, and as words to the participants.

Visionaries have seen lightbody beings and experienced the lightbody phenomena in the lightbody world. This means being taken out of normal reality and put into lightbody reality where lightbody becomes part of the experience. The senses are open. The person experiences the lightbody realm. This includes greater degrees of awareness. The sensitive individual is able to detect the lightrealm influences.

With greater time in the lightbody realm, the individual is able to gain sensitivity to the currents between objects, people, and places. These experiences lead the individual aspirant or apprentice in learning the lightbody knowledge. They have an ability to go beyond their own understanding. They are continually amazed by the experiences they are being opened up to.

It is like a child learning for the first time, experiencing a new place, a wonderful new place. These places are best explored with the master or the teacher. These places are a realm in which the apprentice is learning, but has to be careful not to rush into the traffic. They find themselves in strange and wonderful places. The doors of reality open through space and time for the lightbody traveler.

There are many extreme experiences that the lightbody person or adventurer will want to re-experience. That is possible because lightbody teaching is imprinted within the mind, body, psyche, and lightbody of the participant. One can remember, even though one may not remember.

The process of developing lightbody enhances the ability to see or to be lucid in many ways. This consciousness is one that has to extend from normality to a higher place where one is practicing lightbody techniques or lightbody technology.

Time has to be set aside for the specific manipulation of your mind to go to lightbody realms. Lightbody is not a normal place. Lightbody is a place that can occur in normal reality. It can occur in just a certain small area.

Lightbody is a miraculous thing. We might call it a place and it is energy. It is a manifestation of the spirit that is within our body. Some call it our soul. It is all part of what is identified with the lightbody. The lightbody within us is an identical reflection of who we are.

As we project ourselves and duplicate ourselves into the world of lightbody, we can have that connection with that lightbody and have that dual reality realization. One needs to have a consciousness that goes beyond regular consciousness when splitting ourselves in the lightbody realm. One must do dual duty with one's mind.

We must maintain where we are in our physical body. We must maintain all the conscious functions in keeping that realm together as we travel in the lightbody realm and do lightwork. We are required to take special care of our physical bodies as our missions become more complicated in the lightbody realm. The physical body must not be exhausted, depleted, or go through changes that make work harder, difficult, or impossible.

Lightbody in itself is a special technique, a special procedure, and a special frame of mind that allows the participant to go to other realms. There are limitations. There are warnings or chal-

lenges that are faced by the novice or apprentice in the unfoldment of their lightbody abilities. That is why the teacher-master
has to take the apprentice and give them especially high-level
training in a short amount of time. This training has to be done in
a controlled environment so that other things such as normal life
do not divert the student. A retreat is especially admirable as a
place to do this. A three, four, or five-day retreat to learn lightbody is especially desirable.

There are all forms of lightbody training. The most basic
forms of training involve the knowledge of using the aura in play,
love, sex, healing, and family. All these are connected though
they may seem a bit unconnected. The lightbody experience is a
total experience, a total mind-body-emotion and sexual experience.

It involves devotion by the lightbody players to live in lightbody, relate in lightbody, and have a lightbody community.
Lightbody communities are connected by their lightbody love.
Lightbody love extends between individuals and allows them to
move together in harmony with their mutual love purpose. The
love purpose shared within the lightbody community is magnified
within the lightbody family. The lightbody family includes the
mother, father, and the children together in their relationship.
This builds towards the whole clan, community, or tribe.

Other lightbody relationships are possible with extended families and other alternate love-lifestyles, except that the lightbody
lifestyle is a difficult one to follow. It is one in which the participants, or couples, or families must have a special devotion to each
other that goes beyond mere relationship. The intense intimacy
of lightbody relationships leads individuals to need to be more
than just partners or couples and families.

The lightbody challenge is about people growing and knowing what their future is and what their future is together. Their
lightbody community can help them. Lightbody education is part

of sharing this knowledge and becoming all together higher and more expressive beings.

We share the same space and time and we need to share the joy as well. Harmony will prevail if people can learn to agree, to share, and have compassion. That means to share the healing and the joy.

Applying harmony with destiny is an individual responsibility. It is dependant on the individual's awareness of their place in the universe. What path can they take to get to the fulfillment of those duties? The duties are encompassed not only with one's body and responsibility for its maintenance, but the bodies of those in one's family, community, and world. The role of people when they find their true purpose in life is the true role that they want to play. The play they want to make is the role that they want to be in. That role is the role of being themselves in relationship to others in general. Other relationships include a family group, a tribal group, a lineage group, a national group, and religious groupings.

The role of intimacy in determining the future is of paramount importance. The role of intimate relationships is very important to the future of humanity. The destiny of any person or people, family, or relatives you might know, is important. In this world, and in general, our relativity is so expanded now that we know that we are all interrelated. Our responsibility to many has become paramount to the few, and to those who are aware. Although all should be aware, sometimes there are only a few.

Those who are aware must help all of those who are not aware to become aware of the responsibility of being in the here and now. Those who are not must do what they can to be part of what we are all together. Individuals must do what they will and be what they can. They must take each moment for what they can and do with it what they will. There is a purpose and a way. There is a way through purpose. Everyone has the will to do their purpose and a way to do their will.

We have many bodies that we are already responsible for. All of those bodies are connected to us. We cannot ignore them because we are connected to them to some degree. By taking that connection and going to the next level we can see that we can lift ourselves and lift everybody else. We automatically have in the universe the individuals that we know and love, those that we need to love and maybe forgive. We become better so that we can share the future together in a healthier manner. This means expressing our own individuality and creativity through the medium of our lives and the giving in our work.

As we enjoy the other part of our life, which is possibly not as easy as it should be, we must remember that in our total plan as people we are part of the flow. We are part of families and we are part of forever.

As we go through time and space we end up where we are. This is all part of a loop of where we are going to where we have been. We have already been everywhere anyway. Forever begins with a moment and that moment is forever. It stretches on and on and on, and back and back and back and makes a loop as one makes a loop. The thing is that your loop is not just your loop. Your loop is part of the whole loop. This is part of the whole of humanity. You are part of your family, your clan, and your genetic history. Your genetic history goes back through your mother and father, your family, all of their mothers, fathers, grandmothers, and grandfathers stretching way back.

We do not know who we are going to be related to in the future. We may have an inkling, because we are here and there too. Taking the loop of consciousness through the ride of time allows individuals to see their place in space-time. One is already in realization of where one has gone. One has already been there though one may not have lived it yet. It may be in the future, but one can experience it in the now. One may have experienced it in the past.

The individual has a responsibility to take their own life in their own hands to be part of this flow of eternity. The flow of eternity is in an individual body or entity that takes responsibility. The individual must look after their own well-being and take steps to learn how to sustain their reality. They must know how to sustain themselves, their family, community, nation, world, and environment. That includes the air and space.

As we go through time together, we may not share all the same goals on national, cultural, or religious levels. We are all part of the same flow to wherever we are and to wherever we are going. We are here now. We are here to learn together, to go where we are going together, and to go as individuals.

We have ended up in this space and time. Sharing is the reason we are here. The theme of sharing is to connect. That means not only connections through the body and the mind, but also through the soul, through the spirit, and through time. The lightbody experience is one that stretches into time.

We connect through our consciousness. Consciousness is dependent on thoughts. Giving thought to the connection allows people to go to steps or to plateaus that are enlightening and revealing of the world and the universe at large. Consciousness allows the individual to stretch that far, to stretch that way, and to stretch through time, as they have never seen before.

What an individual is able to do is to become more. They are everybody that they are ever going to be and ever were. Not only that, they are related to everybody who they ever were and ever will be. Everybody is so connected that not knowing that connection is great ignorance. It is something we have ignored because of the necessity of having to pay attention to reality. Reality in itself is a compelling force and factor. By taking steps to harmonize oneself with reality one can become more than an individual. One can become a player in the future.

We have seen the past. We can go there and do things there. The future is still ahead. That is why it takes individuals with foresight and creativity to take the steps that involve using their own force of consciousness. They may have to develop this through their own effort. They might get some training here and there. It requires a great effort and a great devotion. Many choose religion. Many choose prayers to God. Some choose paths to God that are quite difficult.

Some paths are very easy. Some take years to master the procedures. There are others that do not take that much time. It is a matter of devotion. Some people are naturally touched by the energy and are naturally inclined to be religious, intellectual, or physical. All of these are different aspects of how an individual might fulfill themselves at any particular time within their lifetime, within their lifetimes to come, and in the past.

Drawing upon all of one's experiences at once is a difficult challenge for anybody. To do that simultaneously is one of the pleasures of having 20/20 vision in both directions. Not only that, one must have 20/20 vision in all directions. All directions of dimensional space and time can be seen.

That gives an individual a unique vantage point. One is occupying the space and time that one is in. Where is one's vantage point in space-time? Maybe it is between one's ears, or at the third eye, in the heart, or wherever one has managed to place it.

There is a place there that one has chosen to claim. In that position one can challenge oneself to say, "I want control of a little bit behind the eyes," or wherever one pleases. One actually, as a soul and as a spirit, has to claim the body. One has to already be in there and do whatever one can do to keep unwanted beings out of there. That means that if one is getting too influenced by this or that, one has to ask, "Is this or that influencing me too much? Am I listening to the wrong inner voices? Have I heard things that have left me in disarray? Am I actually figuring things out or is it done for me? Am I in control of me? Am I in control of my body and my time?" One has to take the challenge.

That is the most important factor in life. If one has control of one's time, one can say, "I have been in control of these many hours in the day." One can congratulate oneself on that. If one cannot say that, where is one going? Well, one can start with a few minutes at a time and go from there.

What this all means is that those people that have control of their time, space, and life are effective at being channels. If they are not, they are ineffective. They are being channeled through others or by others to do the other's bidding. That may be the right thing if one is in a family. A family group needs to work together and do all that. If one is being manipulated by outside spirits then one has to take control of that situation.

This may not seem like a big problem, but it actually is. There are many people that are visited by spirits. They become possessed by them. Their thinking is changed or molded by spirits that may not have the best intentions and may be using them.

One of the worst problems of power and connectivity is that one starts connecting with everything and being very sensitive. One might be sensitive to the wrong kinds of spirits. The thing about being sensitive to the world and to the universe is that it is all out there. It is not just taking the good and the bad. One cannot just take the good and the bad. There is no such thing as taking the good and the bad. One has to make a choice or else become confused. There are many confused people leading confused nations. The point is not to be confused.

The point is to have the power to control what we might call destiny through intention. It is the power the individual gains through taking control. This may be done through mental exercises, learning concentration, meditation, spiritual exercises, prayer, or any number of methods that give people that ability. Education is the first step.

One way to learn is to first learn to do something and then do it over and over, if necessary. If one needs to continue to do something, then continually do it. Do not ignore that one has to do it, because it needs to be done. If one knows that it needs to be done, and if there is something keeping it from being done, one has to ask oneself what it is. Am I making the decisions? Is someone or something else making the decisions? These are some of the first tests that one has to face, particularly in seeing so much of the universe. If one connects to forces in space and time, and connects their identity to places in space and time, then one might be vulnerable to anything.

It is as if one is a child out there. There are spirits that are like con people out there. They try to confuse and take advantage saying things like, "Let's be friends. You have to do it my way. You have to obey me and do this and that." There might be trouble if it is a sinister spirit. There is much trouble going around. Those seeking spiritual experience may first be warned. There is bliss and ignorance. Sometimes it gets out of hand. One might observe people getting whacked out living abnormal lives.

Observe people. There is a big percentage of unhappiness when people are not following their true path. Maybe they have somehow veered off that path. They may not feel they are where they should be. Maybe it is the environment. Maybe it was wrong choices that they made or were made for them. There might be a way for an individual to reconnect with their life and time in space-time. They may be able to right the wrong that was done against them. Maybe they have done wrong to others. Maybe they wrongly forced their will. They can ask for forgiveness and forgive too. We are to forgive and to ask for forgiveness if needed and necessary. We can get through difficulties even if we need to ask for help in doing that. It is something that is part of the learning process. This is something we can do to help others too.

If one gets that help they know what help is. One knows what help does. One knows what help can do. One knows how and what to do to help others because of having been helped. If one has to help oneself at first with a self-help book or self-help recording, it should have something to do with where one is going. One may have to reject it as false. In looking at that, one can make decisions and go from there.

In the performance of lightbody missions, one usually has to use lightbody powers. The lightbody manifestation is caused by lightbody imagination or by the lightbody willpower that is manifest by willpower. You are the person that is using yourself as the controller of your lightbody.

Lightbody manifestation is a personal manifestation that occurs when a person can use their lightbody to manifest their own will. Being a manifester of lightbody ability, the lightbody apprentice normally has the ability to do things that are mischievous. These should be avoided at all cost because the consequences are severe.

Lightbody knowledge is such that it is grouped in factors that are exponential and can be comprehended exponentially. As the lightbody person learns things, they learn things better and better and better. The magnitude of knowledge becomes greater and the access to that knowledge becomes greater. The entire experience becomes greater.

It is only compassion that brings lightbody masters to teach their apprentices how to experience all of this. The lightbody masters go through such difficulty in teaching the apprentices because the apprentices have no idea what they are about to find. The apprentice can cause the lightbody master so many problems. The lightbody master is at first vulnerable to all kinds of problems just by being a master and being vulnerable to having students. It is too much work for some lightbody masters to take on apprentices. Being a lightbody master involves more than just a single professional position. It may seem to be only one profession, but it is more than one profession. It is a way of connecting all. It is connecting the people that are within one's community, one's clan, and one's family to the lightbody lineage. The lightbody lineage is one that one partakes of because of birth in a lightbody and a physical body.

One enjoys lightbodyhood. Lightbody is a way of being. Lightbody is a way of mind. Lightbody is a way of emotion. Lightbody is an attitude. Lightbody attitude involves manifesting a resonance with the universe. Being in lightbody mind means one is in lightbody. Being in a physical body is a good start. Having one's lightbody in one's physical body to manifest lightbody is the prime purpose of learning the lightbody teaching.

Manifesting oneself on elementary lightbody levels involves using oneself as the lightbody antenna, lightbody conductor, lightbody being, or lightbody entity. The lightbody is an active component in the lightbody world. By being a lightbody you are a lightbody component.

The lightbody world has an attribution list and hierarchy that can be known from literature and particular cultural traditions. Cultures placed different significances on lightbody manifestations that usually were based on their historical connections to certain light entities. Cultural traditions, legends, and politics play a large role in this lightbody hierarchy.

Lightbody technology is one that surpasses regular worldly affairs. Lightbody technology is one that surpasses normal consciousness. It is more than normal consciousness. It is not something one would say is consciousness unless one has it. Because it is something more, it becomes more consciousness.

The expansion of consciousness by using the lightbody is just natural. Using the lightbody is natural. Focusing oneself into being oneself is natural as well. What you find when you are not yourself is that you may have too many blocks to be yourself. You are naturally yourself. Your lightbody wants you to be you.

You can be yourself by being closer to your lightbody. Your lightbody is the blueprint of your life. Lightbody is the pattern you were born with. Lightbody is the structure of your spirit. Lightbody is the identity that is all that is you.

Lightbody Activation

The teacher or master can perform lightbody activation at a distance by using lightbody surrogates or lightbody coordination. Lightbody coordination involves coordinating one's lightbody, if one is the master, to the lightbodies of the apprentices. This can be done with one apprentice or multiple apprentices at one time.

The lightbody activation sequence allows that multiple people in a room or environment can be activated simultaneously. The consciousness of the master has to be connected to all apprentices at the same time. The master has the ability to perform the lightbody activation sequence simultaneously on multiple participants, which is best for mutual and group activation.

Group activation gives the power of the group more power because it simultaneously occurs in all the participants. Activation sequences have a more profound effect when they are harmonized. Having an exact sequence in a group is not absolutely necessary if they can harmonize at a later time in the activation meditation or exercise sequence.

For instance, through use of the master's lightbody, the master activating an individual would be able to, in a first method of activation, go to the apprentice's physical body and lightbody at the same time. The master can perform the activation in various parts of the apprentice's body, usually starting with a general activation of the entire aura and then an activation of what is particularly necessary to activate. The hands are usually activated for the purpose of healing through the hands if the apprentice is a healing apprentice.

The healing sequence for the hands is such that the fingers and the palms of the hands are all activated. Then there is a complete activation of the energy fields within the hand, within the arm, and the entire body as well. Normally, the focusing is on the hand itself. It is important that both hands are activated.

The hands of the apprentice are activated by lightbody activation during the activation sequence. This means that they are imprinted with particular codes that allow them to do lightbody healing. These codes allow the lightbody user to use them as if they were tools, surgical tools, and other types of tools.

In the activation sequence of the individual apparatus, the lightbody master will use their own lightbody to open up portals within the hand area of the apprentice to allow the apprentice to have the access to the tools and the codes.

Then the knowledge procedures are imprinted through the knowledgebase in the third eye. Though that is a separate activation, it is part of the activation of any area such as the hand. The hands will have the knowledgebase within them once they are activated. It is not necessary to know what is going on or what is actually occurring.

The hands have their own ability to use the knowledge. The knowledge is independent of the hands, independent of the lightbody, independent of the physical body, and can even be independent of the mind.

The knowledge carries with itself a power. If the user, master, apprentice, or others who come across it are not careful it could actually use them. In this there is always the danger of becoming overpowered by the knowledge and the old analogy to the Sorcerer's Apprentice is apt in these circumstances.

The knowledge codes that are involved are imprinted in the apprentice and allow them to become an instant master of healing technologies. If they are connected through the third eye, psychic, and other telepathic means, they will have access to libraries of information that are stored within them.

The information is not outside. It is inside and stored within another dimensional framework. The framework is within their domain. It is locked. Seals and codes secure it. Even though this is a secure technology, it is a transferable technology. The activation of the technology is such that it is nondenominational. It has an ability to be manipulated by people of any faith or non-faith really, because of its pure scientific or realistic application.

Modern science might call the lightbody an imaginary, or non-physical body that is possibly unobservable. Someday there may be new instruments that allow the observation of the lightbody.

The lightbody relationship between an individual apprentice and their lightbody can be as if they are very friendly or an even more intense personal identification. The difference is that you can have your lightbody, but your lightbody may have you too. It may go both ways if one is not in control of oneself and in circumstances where the lightbody has a mind of its own. Then the individual in the physical body would have to wonder why.

In the apprentice's struggle to become conscious and activated, they must know and learn what their lightbody is. Through the training that the master provides, the apprentice is able to master the knowledge of lightbody and the use of lightbody in the dangers of the lightbody realm. This is why apprenticeship takes time, whereas enlightenment may not.

Enlightenment and illuminations may occur spontaneously after activation by the lightbody master. The lightbody apprentices have a responsibility to maintain their own dignity, awareness, and ability to learn through this process. Many things could easily divert them.

Lightbody Lessons

To see your lightbody and to learn from your lightbody is to learn the real tough lessons and to learn about your weaknesses. If your lightbody is true to you, your lightbody will show exactly where your weaknesses lie. With most people the weaknesses is not in their conscious mind, but in their unconscious mind, their sleeping mind, or when they are the least prepared.

Most of us can stand up and face problems when we are fully able to. We can stand up to ordinary problems and they are not going to bother us. How well can we stand up to temptations, spirits, or lightbody threats? How well can we stand up to a threat when we are incapacitated, asleep, intoxicated, satiated, or when we are put to the extremes of emotion or of stress?

All of these things may have bearing on our lightbody consciousness and on our physical actions. Emotions and other factors play upon our decision making. Looking after the lightbody is important. One of the most important things that can be done for your lightbody is to look after your lightbody health. Your lightbody health is going to keep your physical health in order.

Your lightbody knows what your physical body needs. Your lightbody makes your physical body happen in a magical way. They call that life. The magical part of the lightbody is its ability to manifest. A natural energy within the lightbody, which is what we call light or energy, is formed with spirit and love. These things combine in the formation of a system of interaction. We call this life when taken to the highest extent. We call this lightbody cooperation.

We find lightbodies in unison working in groups because of their genus or hierarchy. For example, angels are a certain class. The saints are a certain class of beings as are regular people. In looking at the entire realm of spirits we can see that there are different types of spirits that are classifiable by their attributes.

74

Knowing about them is part of knowing the entire spectrum of lightbody.

Part of understanding the resonance between two entities is to understand the classification of the attributes. Are they mammal, animal, or spirit of some sort? There are many possibilities in the basic relationship of one to another. That is how we will go beyond the basics and learn psychic communication. How will we transmit information between the teacher and the student, the master and the apprentice, and so forth?

With that in mind, and taking the basic structure that has been given, we are going to go into the basic relationships. These are between teacher and student. Eventually they are between student and student. There are other forms such as student to non-student. The preparation of the individual student and teacher through time achieves harmonic resonance with others that are working on the same path, or not working on it.

Because of the complexity and nature of this exercise, confidence is required. Strict confidence is sought. What is available is contact with the teacher. The usual form of the format is in the classroom, in person-to-person consultation, or telepathic.

All of these involve great karmic risk to either party involved. The bond between the student and teacher or the master and apprentice can be greater than what is normal in relationships. They are usually longer lasting. The consequences are so great that one has to beware of participating. Such things as these are normally reserved for family, because in those cases the intimacy of the relationship is bonded by blood between those involved.

The first look at the intimacy of the relationship of entity to entity through family allows the transmission of knowledge that surpasses normal means. It is part of the makeup of the individual that inherits certain traits and has connections to certain lineages of psychic beings that visit. This involves an amount of interplay and interchange with the past. Spirits of relatives and spirits that are associated with places, times, and spaces are part of this.

In the learning process, the teacher and the student are able to exchange energy and information because of an agreement. This is usually made for the fulfillment of a certain skill. The skill set that is communicated by the psychic master will determine the skills that the student receives.

The student may try to attain greater heights by following more advanced procedures that are available to the diligent and perseverant student. There are many pursuits available to those daring to take the risk. The dangers are such that one might be influenced too much to be in the normal reality, as we might say, for the required amount of time.

Using these types of energies are usually limited to the scope of the classroom and particular times. That allows the participants to use their energy in a way that does not exhaust them. It does not take too much time out of their schedules or consume their thoughts and mind.

The student's pursuits must be limited to certain exercises and homework. They are only supposed to be done at certain times in coordination with their teacher or master, depending on the complexity of the work.

Normal lightwork would not require a master to teach yet. A teacher might be able to handle the basics. For advanced psychic work it is necessary for the master to teach an apprentice that is fully committed to the path of knowing and being. Unfortunately, there is not much going back. The deeper one becomes, the deeper one is. It is like a sea you jump into. There is not much shallow water. There are many places in which the student and teacher can go together.

There is a great complexity in these relationships that can transcend normal relationships. It is more intimate than most people can realize. The intimacy is such that the harmonics between the teacher and student must be close. The teaching process occurs so that the minds of the two become merged in certain manners. This allows the student to sometimes know more than they should, and many times more than they could without extra help.

When learning from a master, your education may be accelerated to such a degree that you must keep track of how fast you go. How fast can you go? Where are you going in that process? Knowing what you are going to do in the process is essential for the teacher. It offers the student an insight into what they are working towards.

Having an idea of the entire course and the course outline is essential. To follow a procedure of learning allows the psychic to develop skills in an orderly manner and to achieve what their potentials might be.

In the organization of the time spent between the teacher and the student, master and the apprentice, the individuals must know exactly what they want to do and accomplish within the time frame. If they can accomplish more, then they can go to higher levels within the time frame they have.

There are often many consequences of these lessons that extend out into normal life. It is a matter of getting to know what these kinds of experiences bring into the mind and consciousness. When taking this training or learning, it sometimes changes people to such a degree that they must constantly readapt to the world. This is good in a way, yet it is very time-consuming.

What you knew is not true when you know it is changing all of the time. You change all of the time and your perception of time changes too. You become a player in reality instead of a pawn. You are able to do things that everyone is not able to do.

Knowing what your potential is great, yet knowing your limitations is greater. Knowing how to see what needs to be done is part of intuition. It takes an amount of prying and planning to get a good impression of how you can accomplish what you wish.

Doing all one has to do according to a plan is easier than saying, "I think I can do all these things." A random order might be good for some who like to dip and change and find their heart in everything.

People will find it of value to pursue these courses with steadfast attention. Over time this would bring a great discipline to the body and mind. It brings an ability for the person to take their life in their own hands and become more than what they think they are. They can become more of what they think they could be. The future extends from your right now. Your love extends from your heart. Your mind can extend on, too.

What you might see in this training is that you are more than you thought you might be. This is because you are not just a placeholder in reality. You are a player in what is going on all around and within yourself. You have an ability to sense more, to be more, and to have more, or maybe have less. There is the consequence of doing things wrong. Yet, there is greater joy for those who do things right.

Extending the self from the self-within to the self-without is part of the teaching of the lightbody reality. The lightbody reality is an extension of the body, from the body, into the world. The extension normally known as the aura is an extension of the body, as we know. In our aura are energies that we may know and not know, see or not see. There are many things that may lurk there.

Some things are good. Some things are bad. If we look at an aura photograph we might see that the aura in and around the body has a certain glow or emanation. It has colors that are associated with frequencies and can be translated through special cameras or computer programs. We can analyze the information to know what is going on in the aura. We may not understand exactly because there is so much more beyond what can be shown.

In this teaching between the teacher and the student, there is an amount of interaction occurring within and without. This

78

interaction causes a psychic cording between the participants. This is a connection between the minds and bodies of the teacher and student. This allows the connection to become so strong and go so far within that it changes the reality of those involved, the teacher and the student.

In the instance of this teaching there is an inner connection. There is an inner connectivity that can achieve harmony and transmission of information that exceeds the imagination of the student. The information can be complex, but transmitted so efficiently and so immediately that the student has little choice, but gulp. Oh, Wow! It is such a great experience to know more than one did a moment ago, and not have to work so hard for it.

To understand it and unpack it may take a lot more learning. One has to know exactly what happened in the flow that got planted in the mind. One might see the information that is packed there as a database. That applies to knowledge everywhere.

There are methods and procedures to get to know oneself. These are methods to know the world and universe around one. These methods and procedures that we are going to explore now are methods that one can do in classrooms. These are exercises to do with a teacher.

Various postures can be used such as sitting on the floor, sitting on a chair, or even laying down in various positions. Yoga positions can be used for this meditation, as we might call it. Those who can do it can use some forms of yoga. To manipulate the body into various positions besides sitting is especially useful. It allows the student, the apprentice, and the master to do various exercises that are beyond the normal simply sitting down. Light-body training can be taught while a person is sitting on a chair, sitting on the floor, lying down, or standing up. Other positions or movements are also used. It can be observed as dance.

It is an interchange of energy between individuals that are in certain positions in relation to each other. One might ask, "What does the position of an individual have to do with where and what is occurring in the actual training?"

Training the individuals usually starts out in a classroom where several students or more are involved, even twenty or thirty students. In the actual training of an apprentice who needs to know special skills that are beyond classroom skills, there is a more intimate connection between the teacher and the student.

The classroom skills allow the teacher to familiarize the students with a great number of peculiar things that start to occur to them and in the world around them. They should not be mystified or baffled by all the strange occurrences that they are just starting to notice. These things may have been going on all along between the scenes without them seeing it. These things may have been going on under their noses without them seeing, knowing, or believing.

Interchange with the teacher is important in these exercises when the students are starting and learning to become psychic. In this interchange we must understand that there is a resonance that occurs. In this resonance there are certain waves that occur. The waves are often dependent on the position of the bodies in relation to each other. If the people are greatly separated at different parts of the world, there is a different communication than if they were just inches apart. Their auras and their energies would have different effects on each other. Their physical bodies, lightbodies, emotional bodies, and mental bodies would also be affected.

The interesting part about this learning is that it can occur in many locations in many parts of the world. The participants do not have to be in the same location. If a cell phone connects them they might be able to do some things that most people could not imagine. This is especially significant when looking at the ability of lightbeings to communicate and do things at great distances. Communicating through phones, cell phones, and other forms of communications technology is important.

The establishing of mutual energy channels is usually difficult. It takes a good combination of teacher and student to do great transmissions. After a while there is a possibility of greater transmission between students and teacher if the students can harmonize themselves. This may take quite a while. It may take up to a year, two years, or ten years for the student to get their life, mind, and being together to absorb the teaching that the teacher has to offer.

In this knowledge exchange, trying to become more psychic, or aware of psychic abilities and procedures, the individual student has to use their abilities in demonstrable manners. This involves actual experience with the teachers in real time training in becoming the psychic they wish to be.

During the channeling process, the student or medium should have a general set of guidelines.

Holding consciousness is very important in every situation during lightbody manifestation. Holding consciousness is a primary exercise. The conscious mindflow should be thoughtful and meaningful. It means to use one's mind and body to coordinate the recording of information in a desired format. Use audio recording apparatus to record the information. Then transcribe it.

During psychic output it is difficult to determine other factors except than the ones requested. Eliminate decision factors that are not part of the equation. Determine the exact coordinates and possibilities of the situation. The synchronous mental action network determines the exact coordinate possibilities. What is the synchronous mental action network? That is how we work.

Depending on the real thought, the thought becomes the reality. The reality is dependant on all the thoughts in attendance to the thought. The attributes are in a hierarchical form. The attributes determine if the hierarchical form is a matter of metaphysical, physical, or logical order.

Determine what the influences are. The determination is the prescription. The synchronous mental action network has the diagrams and formulas for the translation of the data to the visual and logical format.

This is the lightbody technician's dilemma: How do you deal with the details during the mindflow? How can you hold consciousness and deal with the real? Do you know the necessary things to say or do? If it is evident then go to work on it.

There are often different things in store during the psychic output. Be aware of them and be prepared. Be attendant to time. Take precautions against wasting time during mindflow. Manage assets of consciousness efficiently. Be attentive to the psychic situation at every moment.

In the lightbody universe, the lightbody worker is able to manifest healing through enabling the lightbody manifestation of the portals in the lightbodies of the patient or student. In the lightbody transmission of knowledge or healing, the portals must be opened through lightbody transmission.

The transmission usually occurs through portal openings using portal entity diagrams that can be described in geometrical, logical, and metaphysical terms. All of these terms are related.

The next step in understanding how a geometrical lightform universe exists is to know how relationships exist in a geometrical form. This depends on the one, two, three, or four types of relationship to different spaces between entities, such as one, two, three, or four entities, and so on.

All of these relationships can evolve into geometrical shapes and into the sacred geometries that are well described by others. This is a means of consciousness that uses those entities or those means of geometrical structuring to allow abilities in the apprentice and in the master to influence reality in ways. Lightbodies are enabled to do things that the normal body just cannot do.

The normal body influences the lightbody. The mind of the normal body has an influence on the lightbody because it is the willpower of the normal mind that makes the thing happen. The exercising of the lightbody is to do a specific task or mission.

Lightbody technology is not limited to just regular experience. It is a part of daily life, daily communication, and daily interaction with other people, interaction with the universe, interaction with yourself, your dreamself, and your dreamworld.

Lightbody is a pathway that leads you through understanding yourself. You are yourself through time. Time is your lightbody. Lightbody leads you on and leads you through time, because you are your lightbody. To separate yourself from your lightbody is rather dangerous. You can separate your lightbody from your physical body for an extended amount of time depending on the experience of the participant, apprentice, or master.

The ability of the lightbody to travel out of the body means that the body is less attended by consciousness and the consciousness is placed elsewhere. There may be problems with the breathing if the breathing is not attended to. That is why breathing exercises are widely advised in all religions and all practices of lightbody experience so that the physical body remains alive while the lightbody does its work.

Lightbody work is normally educational. The lightworkers extend the lightbody knowledge throughout the individuals within the family, clan, community, nation, and lineage. That enables the lightbody knowledge be passed on through the lineage to the people. It is available to those who need to heal, to be educated, and to do all the things that lightbody people can do.

Lightbody consciousness is not easy to come by. Once one has it, it is hard to avoid. Being lightbody conscious means that your body and your lightbody are conjoined in your consciousness. One has an ability to work with them in a simultaneous manner. That means that you are resonant with your lightbody. That means that your physical body is resonant with your lightbody. That means you can manifest your lightbody in resonance with your physical body.

How do you test that? Use your lightbody as a resonant force in you and emanate lightfield. Or, use the world at large as a mirror of your lightfield. You have a whole range of choices on reflecting yourself and reflecting your lightbody into the world. You do not want to go out into the lightworld and into your lightbody upon a trivial demand. You should know how to control your lightbody. We have certain responsibilities and certain powers that we can call upon. Lightbody gives us the ability to do those things that we need to do. Lightbody is something that can surpass one's ability to be one. One you. One me. One they. One we. We can become all and can come together.

There are lightbody universes where harmony is a pleasure all can share. In this world there is much conflict. Those who ignore conflict can meditate until flowers grow out of their ears. One has to learn to deal with everything. That is why lightbody training involves a lot more than just meditating. It involves lightbody action, lightbody being, lightbody activation, lightbody energizing, lightbody healing, lightbody mind, and lightbody relationships. Lightbody is something that everybody can do if a little training is applied.

Your lightbody lineage extends from where you are to where you will be and all the family that one has and their families. It extends out through time and as people extend themselves across the earth, it will extend there too. As we will extend ourselves out beyond the earth in space, the lineage will be extended there too. Our heritage and our future are tied together by our present. That is all tied together by you and your presence as a lightbody in your physical body.

That is the important significance of your mission. Your mission in your physical body is to carry on these lineages; your lightbody, your physical body, your identity, your culture, your education, all the wisdom that goes into making you and making what will need to be made in the future into what will be. We are making our future by being ourselves now. The lineage, by being in us, is within us. The lineage extends between each of our blood cells, each of our thought cells, and each of our feelings.

Lightwork

Lightbody play and lightbody work are similar except that the lightbody work is part of a mission to be accomplished. It is either given to you or it is something that you choose to do. In your mission as a lightbody worker it may be that the physical problem of a patient needs to be resolved. That would be the mission. The lightbody worker takes what energies they can from the situation. From there they are able to open a portal around the diseased area and do the lightwork to cure the patient.

Lightbody magic is the working of actions, events, or certain phenomena in reality. These are attributable to lightbody phenomena. Lightbody work is the action or effect of lightbody intention to create various effects. Using one's mind in lightmagic has an influence on destiny, time, and space. The gravity of it all is in the willpower of the apprentice, or the master lightmagician or lightworker. Willpower or intent is used in manifestation in the real world and in the lightworld. The lightworker can manifest in various worlds by using various abilities and powers that they learn during their lightbody training.

In this use of lightbody magic, the lightbody worker does a play that is just part of reality. The healing occurs because it is something good. It is right. Something occurs because it should occur. The thing about lightbody is that it can detect what is good and what is not. It is able to separate that because of the vibrational intensity of the lightbody.

The lightbody is able to cause separations of malignancies and other things from the regular tissue and remove it. This occurs in and out of the physical body through the transmission of the diseased tissue into lightbody world and then out into the physical world again where it is expelled outside the patient. The other healing processes that must go on within the patient are continued on the lightbody, but continued in a way that may not be visible to the lightbody practitioner. It is part of the lightbody work as well. As the patient has their body returned to normal reality, the lightbody reality must take an exit and in this exit there may be a sensation of tingling, energy, and warming.

What is occurring is that the healing is taking a hold of, or changing and manipulating the physical reality to fit the light reality. The lightbody image in the individual is the healthy image. The healthy image is used as a template for recreating wholeness or to fix or bypass the problem within the body receiving the treatment.

Lightbody methodologies are varied throughout cultures, the galaxy, and throughout the universe as well. Part of the lightbody technology is an inherent knowledge or understanding of what is and what should be in regard to the patient. This knowledge has to become part of the lightbody worker. For that to happen the lightbody worker has to tune into the world and the universe. They must receive the appropriate knowledge and information from the person that they are trying to heal.

Psychics that have done fortune telling and actually read the person, the aura, or even talk to the guide or lightbody of the person can give information to that person. They immediately know much about that person. It is the same principle that the lightbody healer, the lightbody worker is going to use. They must use that ability immediately to see exactly what is wrong within the patient. They need to know what needs to be done and to do it immediately.

This is such a fast process that it is practically unbelievable. It takes place in a step-by-step procedure that is orderly. It is accelerated in our consciousness so we are not actually seeing the whole thing. If one were watching a lightbody operation such as a psychic surgery, one would not actually see much time go by. There is much time going by because there are many operations going on within the patient.

The healing process is one in which the instruments and healing or surgical procedures are so small that it is impossible to see unless one is looking through the psychic lens into that lightbody reality. Taking the psychic lens and gazing into the lightbody reality allows one to understand what is occurring when the healing occurs.

Lightbody workers use their hands to effect the vibration or the aura of the patient being treated. These manipulations of the aura or the lightfield are usually on the surface. There are many lightworkers that are beginning to use their abilities to penetrate into the interior of the physical body and to provide lightbody healing to internal organs as well. The lightbody physician can detect the entire situation in the body with their hands. They do not actually need to use their hands. They just need to use their mind or consciousness to scan the body of the individual being treated.

Masters use this methodology and other forms of scanning. When scanning their class for the first time, they see everything. The master should know everything about all the apprentices and their levels, their psychic abilities, and their physical abilities. Everything is available to the gaze of the master psychic surgeon.

The psychic surgeon is able to understand what is necessary or needs to be done in the healing and is able to start to change the reality within the being. This means that the actual place, the actual person starts to undergo a change.

This change is something that may give the patient qualms, uneasiness, or anticipation. They sometimes know that something is on its way. What is happening is that there is a lot happening. A whole lot more is happening than we might imagine. This entire process is so planned out down to the detail that one cannot imagine the complexity.

In looking at a particular operation that a surgeon might do in the real world, one sees that one has to cut here, tie there, and this and that. The psychic surgeon has to rely on other means besides those physical means.

What that means is that the psychic surgeon has to do all those things in a very fast manner in another dimension using their lightbody. The lightbody skills of others that are participating are also used to accomplish something in a fraction of a second that might actually take hours in lightbody time.

The lightbody worker is opening that portal so the lightwork can be done. The lightbody worker uses lightbody field to establish the portal. The lightbody worker is able to pull in the energy through faith, strength, and determination that something is going to happen. The faith of all involved is helpful.

The lightbody worker is someone who is able to use all those forces together to manifest lightbody work. Some people call it magic. Some call it a miracle. Some say it is bogus. The lightbody technology is not one to deceive, but one to help. It was not meant as a trick, but as a trade. Lightbody is something that people do as a way of life. It is preserved in the heritage of the lightbody workers. The lightbody workers are physicians of all times. They take the titles, places, and positions of honor.

Through time these men and women have served through their families, tribes, nations, and lineages to help and heal. These lightbody traditions have been shared throughout the world. Though you may not know too many of these lightbody workers, knowing one of them, or some of the best of them can lead to lightbody understanding.

Lightbody understanding of the lightbody world allows the lightbody healer to do things that others not knowing lightbody thinking cannot do. Lightbody thinking is an accelerated form of thinking. It occurs when an individual can place their mind in a lightbody state, in a lightbody world, taking in lightbody information, and transferring it through the consciousness.

This is sometimes called channeling or being a medium. It is to use lightbody information in the oral, verbal, written, or typed form. What lightbody is able to do is transfer information at a particular rate that is beyond the rate of normal consciousness. It is to communicate in a manner that might not be available to the normal consciousness of the lightbody worker.

The lightbody master has control of various forms of mind and consciousness. Because of the limitations of the physical body and variations in hormone levels of serotonin, melatonin, and other chemicals, even the master will not always have the greatest powers in the lightbody world. The individual lightbody worker is limited by their powers, abilities, and the endurance of their physical body.

To project the lightbody into the world is an actual physical feat that takes much energy by the person doing the lightbody work. They are going to be depleted. If they are not healthy and do not have a diet that will replenish this chemical structure within them, they are going to feel depleted. They will not be able to do too much lightbody work.

In fact, exhaustion could kick in soon. What also occurs is that aging occurs too fast. The mind burns out and the consciousness and memory is not able to absorb any more. The entire system becomes clogged up if the body is not healthy.

It is always good to keep the body healthy and the hormonal levels correct. Planning is necessary for these sessions. The person is then able to use their natural body chemicals to do their lightbody work without exhausting the physical body.

Lightbody dance is the ability of the individual to move their physical body or their lightbody in the realm or arena where they are performing their lightbody activities. Lightbody manipulation by the consciousness of the participant, the apprentice in particular, is necessary to effect the actions or tasks that are assigned during a mission. The lightbody aspirant or apprentice is given various tasks in their mission to test their ability to be a lightbody player.

89

Lightbody play is part of the training. It is the fun part. It is a part that in many cultures is part of the children's play. It is something that is naturally ingrained. These abilities are something that have been part of many indigenous cultures and have added influence. Special traditions are associated with this play, with this activity. It is often associated with religious, mythical, and legendary tales, stories, and practices.

Lightbody training can take the form of training on an oral or telepathic level. These training methods are all viable. They are possible because of the great need of the lightbody community to transmit this information.

The lightbody community is the community of spirits that have lightbodies and are aware of their lightbodies. They can use their lightbodies in this great flow of space and time. These lightbody players or these masters of lightbody can use this flow of space and time to accomplish their missions. They go to places in space and time using their minds and their lightbodies.

Lightbody is something that is an actual attribute of the physical body. It has attributes characteristic of the physical body. The mind of the lightbody has to be very coordinated so it is not manipulated by other influences, such as other outside lightbodies or spirits that might have their own intentions that deviate or divert the lightbody of the apprentice.

In this exploration of the flow of space and time, the master has to share with the apprentice various experiences that prepare them for the best and the worst of the lightbody world. The lightbody world is a place where the participants have greater freedom than in this reality.

There are dangers as well that can cause great havoc and especially emotional or mental danger. There is the possibility of having problems such as deep psychological manifestations of spirits such as ghosts, which are forms of lightbodies, and other lightbodies that have prevalence in realms that we may not ever visit by our own intention. In lightbody traveling one would encounter these beings. The teacher or master has to prepare the student to either fight or flee when danger presents itself.

Lightbody technology has tools that the apprentice has to learn to use. These tools allow the apprentice to do more than they would be able to if they did not have these tools. These tools are empowering. They empower the lightbody user to do things that other lightbody users would not be able to do.

These tool sets are parts of sets that are part of the lightbody tradition. These are available to those pursuing the healing modalities, routines, or training. The procedures are advanced. They show the actual ability or the intention of the lightbody healer to affect the physical body through manipulation of these portals in time and space.

The teacher has great control over the apprentice in their encounters with the lightbody world during the training. It is advisable that the bonding between the teacher and the student become so great that the eventual encounters with adverse influences will not destroy the apprentice.

It is incumbent upon the apprentice to promise not to go where one should not go. Knowing a little bit can get one in much danger. Do not go where one should not go once one knows how to get there. It is a matter of common sense. Common sense applies to the lightbody world.

Lightbody players are adventurous participants in this universe. They face dangers that most people will not face. They have an interior reality that allows them to do what they may not be able to do in the reality that their physical body is in.

In lightbody training, the individual is called to use their skills and their discipline to become masters of themselves. Mastery of themselves includes particular procedures, the concentration skills, the meditation skills, the visualization skills, skills of discipline of will, and the use of willpower upon the world, the astral world, the dream world, and the lightbody world. Their degree of mastery of those skills will determine their ability to use those skills in the lightbody world. Those procedures are part of many traditions.

In the tradition that we are learning in regard to lightbody, the training is in the form of using the physical body of the apprentice to control their lightbody. This is done in various actions, exercises, and eventually in missions that they will do with their teacher, and eventually with other students in their class.

Lightbody play is something that a mother and father can start when their child is very young. Children emanate great lightbody emanation when they are very young.

This lightbody emanation is one that can grow stronger through the care and love of the parents. When lightbody children grow and interact with other children, they like to play. Physical play is one form of play. Lightbody play is another form of play that some children do. It is an imaginary play.

Some children make up these games with the so-called imaginary friends who are lightbeings themselves if there are not real people to play with. In this lightbeing world, the lightbeing play is often being done when children are isolated from the regular environment. If they have specific permissions to play in these manners, they play with their lightbody.

There are various non-violent manners to play when playing with the lightbody. In a classroom environment this is seen as throwing imaginary psychic balls between the players in the room. Doing things with the imagination of the psychic players allows constructs in the lightbody world such as lightbody environments, lightbody furniture, and lightbody atmosphere. The lightbody environment ambiance is determined by the agreement of the master and those participating.

Lightbody understanding or being in a lightbody environment with a group of people is like undergoing group hypnosis. Sometimes only a certain percentage of the people are actually going to become involved in that lightbody session.

When the people have the ability to do lightbody at various degrees together at certain levels of competence, they can make up lightbody pods. These lightbody pods allow the individual within the pod to accomplish more than they could alone. They have their own lightbody shell, energy, and identity.

This protective mutual alliance allows the lightbody players to play in a way that is fun. These pods need a master's protection in the most dangerous situations. Knowledgeable podmasters are needed. The training for becoming a podmaster may occur during a pod mission. A podmaster is a master of lightbody energy and coordinates the crewmembers within the pod.

Lightbody pods have an ability to allow lightbodies to travel through space and time together. Lightbody travel allows individuals to experience different realities. They share it through their own minds and consciousness individually. They may share the same experience or pretty much the same experience.

The imagery should be pretty much the same. When forming pods, different people go through different mental attitudes in different times in their lives. They might be part of different pods at different times. This affiliation is normally done for certain work and missions. These lightbody pods or groups of pods are able to do those tasks.

These pods can have various names or meanings like a lightbody starship, a lightbody ship, or a lightbody vehicle. These lightbody manifestations of group intention are real. They must be imagined. That means it takes the effort of the master and the apprentice or apprentices to imagine their lightbody pods, podships, and lightships for large groups.

The imaginary play that can go on within these realms is immense. The beginning play allows the lightbody student to start to learn how to use lightbody. It is something simple. An example would be using the lightbody to try to influence someone else's presence or aura.

Lightbody exercises can be started when children are young, but not too young. They should be at least two or three years old because they might not quite understand the game if any younger. The danger is that knowing this technology at a very young age and not knowing the limits of it or the restrictions that others might place upon it may leave the child at a disadvantage or it may be an advantage. It is a toss-up on how young a child can be taught lightbody.

In my experience of teaching lightbody, I found that youngsters are able to master these skills to a degree. After the teenage years I did not see much interest in it. Individuals who are very interested in the occult, in using their body energy for personal matters, or means of power, may be interested in lightbody.

Lightbody play is sort of cartoonish in a way if one sees it from a lightbody point of view. People or players are actually using their energetic bodies, their lightbodies to play. In most cases, the player's lightbodies stay within them. In some cases the players are able to expand or retract their aura or different levels of their aura. The powers that are available to the lightbody player are such that they can do things that might be characteristic of superheroes in the cartoon strips.

In the use of these imaginary powers, the lightbody is empowering the person to think in ways they might not be able to under the restrictions of normal consciousness. As one is bound by restrictions that are imposed through education, one faces the difficulty in overcoming restrictions that are not really there.

The use of these lightbody superpowers is especially important in lightbody play. As children grow in learning to use their lightbodies, they can use their lightbodies in manners that are most akin to Eastern martial arts where the actual positions and motions of the body convey lightbody energy and power.

What is seen in these lightbody positions and stances is a lightbody form. This allows the person with that lightbody to assume that lightbody position and form in the lightbody world.

They perform the lightbody action or lightbody magic. What children learn in lightbody play is how to use their lightbody in manners that most children do. This is offensively and defensively. Lightbody games can be passive or aggressive.

From my point of view, being brought up in the tradition of the occult by gazing into crystals, the problem of having to deal with sinister spirits meant learning techniques to protect myself. That is why I developed a system of psychic self-defense.

The other formats or systems that are used around the world do not have to use this basically aggressive form of lightbody play. Most of the religions stress a format of peace in attaining lightbody powers through non-aggressive manners. In this I would not disagree, but I am just offering a different technique.

These techniques are based on psychic warfare and psychic self-defense. They help develop the ability of the psychic player to have confidence. They can go anywhere anytime and defend themselves if necessary and get out of there if necessary.

In psychic play, the psychic players are actually learning defense skills, survivor skills, and skills that will enable them to have power in the real world. These real world powers are attributable to the lightbody. They are skills that allow people to confidently advance with less effort. Some coincidences may be attributable to the use of these lightbody survivor skills.

In more primitive and indigenous societies, the occupations are more limited. The ability of people to assist each other is much easier. Extended families and extended communities allow people to share lightbody experiences. They can overcome problems peacefully through negotiations, compromises, and politics. They rely on grandfathers and grandmothers to come up with the best solutions through the lineage.

What the people are able to do, in certain cases, is to form a bonding that allows people in that group, through their religious practices, to come to the realization of their lightbody abilities. This takes place where their lightbodies can go, the places where

95

they are together as lightbodies in their community, and in their interrelationship as lightbodies. Because of that interrelationship, the people within a lightbody community can sense when somebody is hurt, ill, or not mentally within the lightbody community and could be a problem.

Lightbody consciousness can lead to peace, to understanding of God and of one's place in the world and in the universe. Those trying to attain high spiritual or Godly understanding, connection, and love should find it if they pursue it devoutly. Though it may take time and great perseverance, those things are definitely available to the capable lightbody aspirant.

It is recommended the person who is an apprentice lightbody worker first learn lightbody play. This format of play is like the games that children play. Press or push against someone's aura without actually making physical contact. Push against the other person's aura or lightbody as children play.

The whole process has to be visually demonstrated. What occurs is that individuals, without touching each other, are able to affect each other's lightbody and learn from that. People learn these skills and some people have them naturally. Some people have the ability to use their lightbody to manipulate vibrations, attitudes, or the ambiance of a room. They can even make contact with pets such as cats or wild animals and communicate in ways that lightbody allows.

Some of the first games that a lightbody apprentice would learn would be how to defend themselves from lightbody attacks. These defensive mechanisms or tools are usually defined as shielding. Shells, lightforms, and structures protect the lightbody, or the person and the lightbody, from damage and attack.

Why should you be attacked if you are not out there being mean and attacking everybody else? The answer is, things like that happen. If you are able to attain the higher levels of consciousness and such, then lower manifestations and those things should not bother you. If you have not achieved that state of

96

mind then you may have challenges. Those challenges are best met through being prepared for them. The preparation for those challenges is part of being aware in all of your reality. That means being aware in your mind, in your everyday life, dream life, fantasy life, and lightbody life. When one is learning lightbody, one is learning how to actually be part of many worlds. The person who is a lightbody player is playing in many worlds.

Lightbody sports are sports between players of different groups. The different groups can be of the same religion, different religions, or different practices. The judges, umpires, and other officials of lightbody sports regulate the entire game format. Lightbody sports consist of competitions between individual players and teams of players that use lightbody abilities to accomplish certain game objectives. Points are gained through simple game playing skills using winning strategies. The player who accidentally touches the other player is the automatic loser.

The game most common is the circle game. In this game an individual of one team faces an individual from the other team. Then they try to force the other player's physical body out of the ring without actually touching them by using their auric bodies and lightbody. This is all non-violent. At least there is no physical contact. Make as ugly a face as you like.

The entire process is one of attaining power on lightlevel. Lightbody sports are sports that can be played in the same physical arena or the same area. The lightplayers can be separated by certain distances such as having the physical bodies of the lightplayers at different points in the arena. The actual play is in an area or ring as if it were a circus ring. The competition is judged by lightbody masters who have observed this lightbody play. Lightbody competition shows the strengths and weaknesses of each individual's lightbody practice.

The lightbody marshal arts are some of the most demonstrable formats that can be shown. The other formats such as using lightbody methodology to induce forms of knowledge, enlighten-

97

ment, and ecstasy through lightbody manipulation are explained elsewhere. Lightbody sports are separate from the other lightbody activities. They can be observed by an audience in an actual arena and have physical consequences upon the players involved.

Lightbody sports can be played with a physical audience. Physical players play at the specified distance from each other doing what they can to accomplish the aims of that game. There might be a face off of two players at ten feet apart from each other. They must stay within a ring and try to force each other out of the ring without touching each other. They have no other tools besides their hands and their body. In using only their aura and their lightbodies, their aim is to accomplish positional advantage by overcoming the opponent. They make them yield their territory through overwhelming presence of spirit and accommodation through the help of their lightbody.

The actual training of a lightbody apprentice is one in which the lightbody apprentice has to meet their own lightbody at some point. This is their trainer that is going to be working with them throughout their life. This lightbody may at first show the student what they must learn. This lightbody may scare you. The student may possibly experience a gentle surprise attack from this lightbody as a wake-up call. This lightbody may tickle you. Knowing this being that is trying to be seen or understood by you may be something that you may not understand at first.

You may think that if this is my lightbody, it is like a guardian angel. It should keep the bad things ten feet away. But the lightbody is not something that is off on its own trip. It is trying to help you. In too many cases it is doing all the work. Your lightbody is pulling off miracles right and left for you. You are not even doing your part to keep yourself healthy, protected, and safe. Your lightbody is working overtime, all the time, to keep you in line and out of harm's way. The way the lightbody works is through its love of you, and it helps you to do what you need to do.

Developing Aura and Lightfield

This chapter is about developing aura and lightfield. The exercise involves the group training together. This can be one or more people as students. The teacher will not participate in the exercise, but will supervise and monitor the exercise.

This exercise is based on using the body as a sensing mechanism organism device. In this instance a crystal or a crystal ball is used. It is placed in a location that is central to the participants in the exercise, such as in the middle of a room.

The exercise can use various types of crystals and minerals as the focus. This exercise, the basic one, involves a quartz crystal, preferably of one hundred millimeters or greater size in a crystal ball form. The necessity of having quartz is the main factor. The size does not have to be one hundred millimeters. It can be smaller than that.

It can be natural quartz with the least amount of flaws or inclusions. It does not have to be in the spherical crystal ball form. The ideal is a larger crystal ball preferably made from what is called fused, man-made, laboratory grown, or reconstituted quartz. Glass is not usable. Other substances are not of the same quality of quartz for transmission. One should either have a natural quartz crystal or a fused quartz crystal that has been cut and ground into a spherical shape. A spherical shaped crystal is best for these exercises. Fused quartz has special conductive properties that make it easier to use than naturally grown quartz crystals.

Once the crystal has been placed in position, the participants take their positions around it in a circle. The participants start by facing the crystal ball at equal distance from it. The exercise can be done on the floor with people sitting down or at a table. If a table is used, then be careful. If the table is inadvertently bumped or juggled, the crystal ball might roll and possibly fall, break, or be damaged. That is a consideration. The crystal ball is a fragile precision instrument.

The exercise is a guided meditation. The meditation is a gazing meditation to start with. The participants will use their entire body in the exercise. They will make various hand motions and assume different bodily positions so as to change their reference to the crystal itself. The crystal is the focus of the exercise.

The athletes, auric athletes as we would know them, circle the crystal. If there were four participants, four athletes, they would sit at the four directions in the traditional medicine wheel style. The goal is to develop interchange of energy between the individual, the crystal, and the universe. This is a connective energy exercise.

The teacher will guide the meditation by establishing a distance between the crystal and the individuals participating. The first rule is that the participants cannot touch the crystal ball. Their hands should be well out of range of the crystal. Several inches to a foot are the closest they should get to it.

This is to prevent the energy from shorting out. The participant must not accidentally cause a short circuit between the crystal ball, the participant, and the earth. That would ground out the crystal whereas this energy exercise requires that the participants interchange the energy and not ground it out.

There is a distance factor that only allows a certain number of people at a certain distance from the crystal. If there are more than half a dozen people participating, it is difficult to get them all close enough without touching each other. This would cause shorting out of energy fields. If there are more than six people, then the necessity of breaking up into smaller groups becomes paramount in these exercises.

It is necessary to have other teachers or apprentice teachers able to maintain the discipline within these other small groups. The master teacher has to monitor all of the apprentices, all of the exercises, and of all the energy interchanges.

The participants can assume various seated positions, or even yoga positions. These should be comfortable positions with or without cushions, as they are going to be in various rotations.

When the first exercise occurs in this series, the teacher will have the participants locate themselves at specific positions. These positions around the crystal ball are geometric. If there are two then they are directly across from each other. If there are three then they are in a triangle. If there are four it is a square and so on.

The exercise can be part of a larger group of exercises and tuning exercises. This exercise can come at some point within a regime or schedule of exercises. This depends on the classes being offered and the levels of the participants. Because of its nature, the teacher does most of the guided work until the individuals feel the fields. Then they are allowed to trade places with another student or stand up. The teacher should not sit in a circle during the exercise.

What will occur is that each of the participants will be given a focus, a time to focus upon the crystal with their concentration, their gaze, and their energy. The other participants will monitor and try to maintain balance. This is so the participant has the full engagement with the crystal itself, not the other individuals within the circle. The intent of the exercise should be neutral and not tainted by sexual desires or other distractions. Those can divert participants from the course of concentration and the manifestation of will in this exercise.

The participants are required to have a set of mental qualities. These qualities allow them to be disciplined in a manner that is conducive to participation in the exercise. If the teacher says to maintain an energy connection with the crystal at a particular distance and at a certain frequency and magnitude, then the participant, or auric athlete, will do that until told to change. The energy manifested through the exercise can be small or great.

Normally the participants do various exercise attunements. The goal is to achieve mastery of various forms of the auric interchange with the crystal ball. The timing of the exercise is especially important. The impact of the exercise upon the other participants can be gauged over time.

The nature of the exercise is that once the first circle of the exercise is complete, then the other participants can and will do coordinating exercises. They will be able to interchange energy from distances. The distance energy exchange and cross current energy exchange exercises are part of a greater set and more advanced series of exercises.

The full implication of these exercises is that everyone participating is in harmony or resonance to a certain degree, despite having their particular frequencies. By participating in the exercise in the same room or area, the people are able to interchange energy and have a common intent. The common intent allows them to do things that are out of the ordinary and possibly miraculous. The entire reason for doing the exercises is to achieve mastery of the energy, the fields, and the ideas.

Most of this can come through teaching and exercises. As we get back to the first exercise, the participants will start by facing each other and gazing into the crystal. They try to establish a contact with the energy of the crystal.

The teacher will have previously energized the crystal. It will have been cleansed, energized, and located within the circle upon a neutral cushion, stand, or pedestal. When they are able to establish a connection with that energy, the participants are able to, through a series of concentration maneuvers, find themselves in various states of higher consciousness. They learn various abilities to manipulate the fields between the mind and the crystal.

The crystal itself is a focusing mechanism. The crystal allows the individual to extend and to refocus their energy to a greater magnitude if they are in harmony with it. Manifestation of the individual's energy through the crystal allows the individuals to magnify their own potentials.

The coordination of the energy output through synchronized energy manipulation occurs within a group or circle. This allows the coordination wave effect that is important in establishing a higher degree of energy field manipulation. It follows the path of intent of the participants, especially the master teacher, who is guiding this meditation and these auric exercises.

The extension of the individual's ability into the world through the use of their aura and their lightbody is the reason for doing these exercises. The exercises allow the participant to see and be more of who they are. They must use all of who and what they are to effect the connection and do the energy manipulation that is part of this exercise. The participants may have received previous training in energy manipulation that could be useful.

The energy interchange will initially require the person, participant, or individual, to connect directly with the crystal. They use that connection to transmit various energy formats, at various frequencies and durations. The participants use the crystal as if it were a transmission device, as it is.

The connection can be done through the mind or through the hands. The participant can raise their hand and hold it up or out near the crystal. This should be at least several inches away at the closest, until the energy field is established between the individual and the crystal.

The energy field there is then the key to establishing the mutual resonance and harmony between that individual and the crystal. Other individuals within the group establish their own connectivity with the crystal. Eventually they are able to establish a matrix of relationships together.

Because of the harmonizing nature of the crystal, the master teacher can manipulate the multifaceted vibrational interchange of energy. It can then be harmonized to an even greater extent so that the exercise and participants are on track and follow the procedures as prescribed.

The master teacher will establish a routine of exercises. These allow individuals to grow within their own potential. At the same time it forces them to grow faster by being more aware of what they can do.

The nature of these exercises is such that the participant may not at first know whether they can do it. Just by participating for a short amount of time, the effect becomes prominent or becomes manifest. This is to a certain degree related to the activation skills of the master teacher, who can activate the chakras of the participants from a distance.

This whole process of activation, coordination, synchronization, and establishing energy resonance between the participants and the crystal allows the entire matrix to establish a space-time field. This allows other entities to enter. The participants eventually receive spiritual and religious experiences or trainings from others in space and time.

The portals established through these exercises are important. Therein is the intent of the participants. They are able to establish these energy portals within their own circles and their own spaces and times. The master teaches how to establish space-time portals. Being a teacher of this knowledge is much greater than the understanding of normal individuals. This is an understanding of space and time. It is not easily communicated in words and concepts. The concepts are so great that our minds may not comprehend them without a great amount of training.

Therein lies education's importance in this entire field of study. The master teacher will have responsibilities that extend from the moment the participants activate their own selves in these games, aura athletics, energy events, or auric exercises.

The participants should know that they are establishing portals in space and time through their participation. They can come back to relearn, relive, and re-experience the portals. They can relearn and learn from all that they have done. They can share everything they know with those who would learn it. They become teachers instantly because it is ingrained within them. By remembering and sharing they can become portals themselves. They share the joy and the pleasure of being connected and being a part of the universe.

This all comes back to the energy exercises that the participants are sitting around the circle waiting to do. As they go through these they find that the interchange of energy between the individual and the crystal can be set up. In various routines there are frequency modulations that occur between the individual and the crystal.

Tonal augmentation of the environment with sound such as made with crystal bowls can be used for some exercises. Background music can also be used if it is not intrusive. Lighting is another consideration. Avoid bright lights on the crystal itself.

The participants do not have to see the crystal to participate in the initial exercises. The crystal ball itself has been used for gazing for ages. To use it as an energy interchange device is especially important. It allows the individual gazer to develop the skills that will allow them to do the gazing.

These athletic aura skills are part of the training of the gazer, the scryer, and those that would travel through space and time. The pleasures of doing this are evident to those who venture out into those realms. The adventure starts with the discipline of being within the circle, within the crystal's auric energy field, and establishing contact with the crystal. Those individuals participating will eventually attain their own crystals and their own particular contact with those crystals. They will probably have different energy experiences with each crystal.

The training the master teacher is able to provide is one that is instantaneously absorbed by the participants. It is a field manipulation by the teacher that allows the participants to absorb the teaching within themselves, their chakras, and their bodies.

They become part of the teaching and have the teaching thoroughly within them. Teachers use their own energy manipulation skills to give crystals a frequency resonance. This will emanate from the crystal to establish the learning routines that are necessary for the participant. These are naturally built into the crystal if it is a quartz crystal. Other crystals have their own flavors. Quartz is the easiest to work with. It is preferred because of its organization and its ability to have coordination with reality.

One will find that there are aura shells or energy shells that can emanate from the crystal at different distances. One can observe these by using one's hand or one's mind to reflect from the crystal at various distances. This occurs if there are others placing energy within the crystal to give it a frequency vibration. It is like shockwaves being sent out from the center of the body of the crystal ball. This occurs because of the activation through the energy of the individuals participating.

The crystal itself may not vibrate, but the energy that is emanating from it does cause change. The change is one of organizing energy and fields within its proximity. The higher and the greater the input, the higher and greater the output will be.

The individuals in the exercise will focus upon the crystal. They will attain some resonance and interchange with the crystal. At the direction of the instructor, they will be able to do different types of interchanges. They will learn interchange of energy between themselves and other individuals in the circle at various timings and at various distances.

The whole geometric structure of the circle allows the interchange of energies. Circles are such that there can be a greater awakening or activation that can come through a progressive heightening of awareness. The energy works itself up in a circular spiral and through time raises the consciousness of those that are participating. Their minds may not understand what is going on, but something is occurring.

The underlying factors involved may change their mental and biobody. It may impact their lives. It should organize and give direction and purpose to the participants in these exercises.

The connectivity of the individual with the crystal in these initial exercises allows the individual through that contact to use their ability. They can use their mind to manipulate energy. This prepares them for the exercises. Auric energetic exercises involve individuals and not the crystal itself.

At this point, the exercise can be done with the individuals changing their position to the crystal. They can turn and put their backs towards the crystal. There can feel a different connectivity, such as the connectivity to the chakras on their back at different points.

These exercises are such that the teacher has a great duty. The teacher coordinates mutual and high-energy exchanges between the participants. Because of the inner connectivity and intimacy of energy interflow, it is necessary to have a good harmony between the individuals before doing these exercises.

Because these harmonizing exercises allow such great intimacy of thought and energy, the people and participants may become more endeared to each other. They should already have a certain degree of trust and understanding. They trust that this process will bring them closer together and allow them to work together on much higher degrees and levels of love. They are embarking on an emotional adventure that will take them near and far.

The participants have an obligation not to lose their identities or emotions in the exercises or become overwhelmed by them. The teacher has to monitor the experience of the individuals while they are undergoing this training because it is advanced. It involves understanding. This sometimes stretches the boundaries of the person's personal consciousness beyond what they are normally allowed to understand or do.

Participants may occasionally snap back into a normal form of thinking. This is desirable if they need to quickly get back to reality. If the snap back was involuntary then one would have to go back a step and learn more of the basics before getting onto that level again. The teacher will recognize when certain students need personal training to go farther and advance in other ways.

The participants should understand that their growth is not something that they may see immediately. It may occur in the weeks and the months after the event of the meditation, the exercises, and the activations. These activations are such that they are non-religious and are stepping-stones to higher consciousness. Activations may be religious events. Activations may occur in relation to religious activities such as praying.

The importance of this technology is that it is a neutral mechanism. It is usable by people of any faith, persuasion, gender, or intention. What it is used for is entirely up to those that use it. Those who use it for ill will find ill is used against them. It is more of a tool and it has its own karmic obligations. As we might frame it in the West, destiny is such that one has to do well to receive well.

As the individuals are able to go through these energy manipulation exercises and meditations at certain points, they will feel in communication and contact with the entire universe. This is part of the individual's awakening to the world, the universe, and to space and time. In these exercises the individual will receive greater information than normally allowable. This is desirable for those that are undergoing training in channeling, scrying into the future and into the past for information. Using the crystal ball for doing research into space and time is one of the reasons for getting into shape with these auric exercises and this lightbody training.

The lightbody training is a more advanced form of these meditations. It allows the individual or the scryer to go through space and time to receive the knowledge. They can actually live the event, if necessary, to get the information, knowledge, or the path that is being inquired about. Gazers themselves have the tool, which is the crystal ball. Having the method of using it is within their grasp and takes training.

The training is not easy. It is a form of concentration, of having faith as well, and understanding of what is going on. The understanding can come later. Those without any knowledge of this can gaze into a crystal ball and see.

This is an innate talent that is part of our human makeup, our genetic inheritance, and part of our consciousness. Those who feel attracted by crystals are often also attracted by the energy within them and the energy that might emanate from them.

In the exercises, the individual participant is going through personal growth. This will allow them to connect to the greater whole of space and time. They can become a player in destiny, their own destiny as a start. This connectivity gives the individual a role in manipulating the circumstances and destiny that they are part of.

These exercises will have an effect on the lives of family members and other people in the participant's proximity. There is an amount of growth that has to occur. This occurs when someone becomes more aware, more energetic, and hopefully happier. They will feel full of love and that makes everyone around them happier as well.

The path of a gazer, scryer, and energy-field lightworker takes them through realms that people that are not connected within the healing community would know about. These are types of contact in consciousness that allow individuals to become givers, healers, physicians of nature, and psychic physicians. When a gazer is gazing into a crystal, they can receive advice that heals destiny.

The idea of seeing into the future is a phenomenon of lightbody. The lightbody is a traveler. It is a traveler of consciousness. One lets their consciousness travel where it will travel in the lightbody realm, the lightbody world, the lightbody universe, and the lightbody dimensions. There are parallel dimensions as well that can have possible lightbody futures. Remember there are other gazers out there and other makers of the lightbody futures. As gazers go, only the Big Gazer in the sky gets His will.

The initiation of objects for lightbody work involves using one's lightbody to attain affinity or resonance with the object. This enables the use of the lightbody's emanation potential if one is using a crystal or a crystal ball.

The quality of a crystal ball will now be examined. The crystal size is important, but it does not determinate the amount of energy that can be emitted. The determiner is the amount of spirit available to the lightbody worker. The crystal ball is a magnifier of energies that are available to the lightbody worker. It can be used to magnify intentions and energies in the direction of the patient or the apprentice. The lightbody worker may use the crystal and other devices for their work.

The influence of the lightbody on inanimate objects is determined by the amount of spirit that is available to the lightbody worker. When working with a crystal for the first time, one may not feel much energy from it at all. It takes spirit to energize the crystal. The crystal is energized when spirit flows through the hands of the lightworker into it.

Light energy is delivered when spirit influences the lightworker. The lightworker may experience physical reactions during the crystal energizing. The lightworker may become startled by the amount of energy that their hands or the crystal begins to emit. This energy may invoke involuntary muscular reactions and may surprise the lightworker. Energy shockwaves may be felt as a resonance builds between the crystal and the lightworker.

Light energy is then delivered through the hands of the lightworker. Some lightworkers may have to wait longer than others for this energy to manifest. When the resonance occurs, the energy interchange between the crystal and the lightworker becomes intense. The energy will flow out of the hands of the lightworker. The lightworker's shoulders and arms may also become highly energized and be subject to unexpected spasms. This energy may cause the lightworker to suddenly tremble or shake. The energy may cause the lightworker to jump and shout.

This energy is something that just happens for some light-workers. Not everyone can invoke the spirit energy by saying something such as, "Light on now." It is something that just happens sometimes, but it can happen under certain conditions.

The following energy exercises with crystals can help the lightworker to gain control over his or her aura and lightfield.

Place the hands within varying distances from the crystal. Toy with these energy interchanges. Get a feel for the energy between the hands and the crystal. Learn to manipulate the energy. Lift and move the energy with the motion of the hands. The energy is like water. It can be lifted. It can be splashed. It can be directed. It can be played with. It is as if one were throwing a ball in one's hands.

A meditative procedure may be used to invoke the spirit energy while working with the crystal. The spirit energy will infuse into the crystal and leave a residual intelligence. This allows the recipient to understand what transference of spirit or energy was involved. This is the intelligence of the spirit. This intelligence is available to those that are contacted by the spirit, use the spirit, and are mediums of the Holy Spirit.

To feel an inanimate object's influence and power, the light-worker must find the resonance within their own lightbody. They must feel the resonance within the object that they are working with. This may involve the moving of the hands within a few inches to possibly a few feet from an object such as a crystal ball.

A two hundred millimeter fused quartz crystal ball is ideal for this exercise. The crystal ball should have no inclusions and should be crystal clear. The participant can place their hands at a few inches away on either side of the crystal. One might feel a gentle energy emitting from the crystal. It may feel like a soft breeze upon the fingers. Play with that energy until it grows stronger in your hands. Move your hands around it and feel where its auric shells are. Feel the fields and shells that surround the crystal and extend beyond the crystal. These fields give it auric integrity.

Move your hands farther away from the crystal and notice different energy shells at different distances. Push one hand toward the crystal and pull your other hand away at the same time. Then reverse the energy flow as your hands move to and fro. Move the energy back and forth. Weave the energy with your fingers.

The auric shells surrounding objects are knowable by the lightworker. These shells can be felt and attuned to. The crystal ball is a device, a lightbody device. They can be of various sizes, shapes, and formations in order to give the desired and required frequencies and effects.

A spherical crystal shape will emit spherical shells of auric energy when energized. It has well-known physical characteristics. The distance to strong shells can be determined by mathematical calculations based on the size of the crystal and the energy input.

If used properly, the lightbody worker can use these crystal balls as transmitting instruments. The lightbody worker has to attain an effective affinity with the crystal ball in order to use it for transmission of light energy and effect changes in the other bodies. To attain that affinity, the lightbody worker makes an alliance with the crystal.

Lightbody workers need to learn how to work with the universal intelligence. This is the intelligence of the Spirit. This is everywhere. It is within everything that the Spirit is in. The Spirit is God. It is part of the entire universe. Spirit is part of the lifeblood of the universe. Spirit is the working energy in lightbody technology. Using lightbody energy is using spiritual energy, which is using universal spirit energy.

The manifestation wave and field are related through intention by the parallels in the geometric equations. These are established along the lines of matter, energy, and their relationships to light, antimatter, antienergy, and a constant. Processing and coordinating various energies depends on splitting the consciousness along parallel lines of mutual manifestation. This is done by directing segments of the consciousness to the appendages available such as left arm, right arm, left leg, right leg, head area, eyes, mouth, other organs, and the skin.

There is a purpose for the external and internal manifestation of the coordination through the vehicle of the body in its relationship to the entire field. The purpose of the manifestation dealing with the intention depends on what parallel planes are necessary to coordinate. The physical plane is a plane that humans are involved in. The mental plane is more of an intellectual plane. Other planes can be described scientifically by their frequencies and manifestation of attributes. Space-time coordinates and energy manifestation fields characterize these. They depend on the amount of matter and energy in a particular location or antimatter and antienergy. Particular coordinates in space and time deliver that important information.

That information is classifiable by its attributes. The attributes not only include the positions in space-time, but also the past and the future of those coordinates and energy manifestations. By accessing particular places at particular times and setting up coordinates in an absolute manner, the full potential of the equations are realized.

The manifestation of an individual's aura and lightfield in the normal world shows that they have those capabilities in their body. These fields are similar to the fields of star systems, galaxies, and super galaxies. People have the same capabilities as planets and galaxies if they can realize their own potential.

The manifestation of the energy fields depends on what we would call the chakras and the nadis. The nadis are the veins that convey the energy within and around the body. The amount of energy taken to gain the perception necessary to convert these equations into everyday experience is really not much. Because of the construction of the human vehicle, we are able to convey energy. We are able to generate or invoke it within and without, and from the environment. We then channel it through us and through the environment as conduits of the energy.

The energy itself does not have to be visible or measurable in our terms, such as electrical energy or as materials that have electrical and magnetic energy. By using the space and time that the individual is encompassed in, the individual can be a vehicle for the energy flow of time and event. The individual entity, being or spirit might be identified with what we call a person in a body in our world. People are given names so that we do not lose track of where or who they are. We are also connected with animals and the environment. In a meaningful relationship with the universe, one not only has a connection with the buildings around us, but with the trees, water, ground, air, sky, and all of the planets.

By establishing the connection between the individual and the world we see that the power of the individual is enhanced. Concentration and intention is applied in making the connection between space-time worlds. Connective consciousness means to contact other entities or to contact other spaces and times.

We are limited in the types of energy we can emit. This depends on our body's limitations unless we can use other bodies that we are not normally aware of. These are subtle bodies that are dependant on the body itself. Sometimes they are not dependant. In our case as human beings these subtle bodies are dependant on the physical body if we are in control of the physical body, in control of the mortality of the body, in control of the individual path of the body in time, through time, and in time-space.

114

Lightbody Intimacy

Psychic love is a love that extends throughout humanity. Although it is recognized in various forms, it is the bonding and intimacy that goes beyond the ordinary bonding. These types of bondings are especially common in what might be termed more primitive, natural, or indigenous cultures. The family unit is more tightly bound than in the more industrial societies today. The interchange of time, communication, and experience in family units makes possible a synchronicity of efforts and energies. That makes psychic development easier.

The abilities gained by being in a family, especially a psychic family, are widespread and are useful survival skills. These are useful skills for relationships, which are interconnected as well. The connectivity that psychic relationships offer is much greater than mere verbal communication. It is akin to animal communications that are not always based on various sounds made by other members of the same species or evidence of behavior patterns such as movements that are recognizable to other members of the species.

What arises or what is evident in the psychic family is a bonding of love. Through time and genetics and all kinds of experience together this bond builds between the individuals starting with the love between the parents before they were parents. The entire structure of love within a psychic relationship is one that is not isolated to the individuals in love. The individuals in love and in a relationship, especially if they are young, have the ability to have children and procreate for the furtherance of their lineage. At that point they are joining their lineages in their relationship of love.

Love is a fact and factor in the uniting of various lineages. The millions of lineages that are now evident in the world at one time were fewer. The interconnection between lineages is strong, although as individuals we may not see that today in our present tense.

Knowledge of the lineage and the past is always inherent in what we do as individuals. Relationships, especially when in marriage or contemplating marriage, are not just the union of two people, but are the lineage union. There is so much that comes together in this point of marriage, for it continues through space and time.

These relationships are nexus points and they have great power. The individuals in these relationships have great responsibilities, much more than to whom they think they might be at the moment. There is more than lust and love influencing their momentary decisions. There may be much more happening that is influencing them in one way or another.

The establishment of relationships for propagation of the family and the species is the purpose of life, human life especially, and all living creatures on earth. Many or most of them have biological urges that attract them to the opposite sex. Those urges, instinctual and otherwise, stimulate their procreative process and stimulate inclinations for experiences or relationships.

When considering the place of the individual in their relationships to others, the psychic component becomes especially important. When choosing a mate, a life-long mate, there are certain advantages of having a psychic mate. A psychically harmonized mate has, in other words, joined you.

There are many ways to try to figure out who is the right psychic mate. A psychic may intuitively know whether a couple's future together is going to be good. The couple might have visionary experiences or deep feelings about positive experiences ahead together in the real world. The couple may have common goals and feel that they can have pleasure together, work together, and live together. These are pre-requisites for any serious romantic relationship.

We want to discover the difference between a regular relationship, a regular romantic relationship, and a psychic relationship. The psychic relationship has various components or attributes that allow the couple, and eventually their family and extended family, to have greater intimacy. Why would one want greater intimacy? That is the goal of this pursuit of psychic love and psychic sex. Psychic intimacy is all connected and it all deals with family connections. These kinds of family connections are through the physical body, through relationships, through mother, father, children, brothers, sisters and relatives. All of these people are connected through the genes and should be connected through love. Events sometimes create difficulty in that.

In examining lightbody intimacy one sees an entire realm of lightbody relationships that have certain characteristics. Morals and ethics are always involved. Dignity and respect are paramount. Lightbody ethics and morality is a large topic. It involves the faith, religion, and practices of the individual.

There is an entire school in each religion on how to relate to one's partner, one's marriage mate, in a lightbody manner. The lightbody intimacy is able to extend into that relationship and becomes part of the social structure and family connectivity. The intimacy on a certain level is a personal intimacy between two lovers. The love created by this intimacy may cause a new couple to want children and an extended family. This intimacy is just the beginning of greater intimacies and pleasures. This kind of intimacy extends to the ordinary experiences that family members share together such as during meals or praying.

Lightbody intimacy between two lightbodies is a beautiful experience. That is best accomplished through understanding the process of intimacy in the lightbody realms. Lightbodies are like physical bodies and they also have other attributes that physical bodies do not have. Lightbodies do not have physical attributes that the physical bodies have.

In separating these sets of attributes we can say that the lightbody is not a physical body, though it is a body that might be characterized as having physical characteristics. The lightbody has the shape of the physical body. In most cases the lightbody is molded or based on the body of the physical manifestation. This is what the lightbody, or the soul, or spirit of the body chose as their manifestation vehicle, or their expression of identity.

The body system that allows individuals to achieve intimacy is based on resonant harmonies within the lightbodies themselves. In the activation of intimacy, the lightbody participants need to come to agreements. These agreements allow interchanging of energies. The first agreements are physical agreements, meaning that the people in the physical body agree to have some realistic interaction. This is the most basic form of initiating these types of intimate relationships.

There are other intimate relationships that do not involve physical contact at all. Lightbodies have freedoms to do various actions in the lightbody realms and have intimate experiences in those realms as well. Lightbody relationships can occur between people who do not actually know each other in the real world. Many people would remember these lightbody experiences as dreams. Some would remember them as visions, fantasies, or daydreams maybe, but not quite. These intimacies in the lightbody realm are realistic. Some people experiencing these phenomena may think of it as lustful voyeurism and excursions into fantasy.

In many ways there are more connections and much more happening than meets the eye. Intimacy on these lightbody levels has many formats. Let us begin with the first format, which is the format of two individuals who have agreed to have lightbody intimacy. In this lightbody intimacy exercise, the physical bodies of the participants can be separated by any distance, but for practical purposes being in the same room or adjoining rooms is OK.

It is possible to have individuals participate in these exercises at different times, or in different time zones, but the complexity makes it much more difficult. That is more in the abilities of the lightbody masters than apprentices. In real time lightbody intimacy exercises, the individuals will probably be in the same room and be in a comfortable seating position or lying down.

In most cases, because of the intimacy of this exercise, the intimacy does not extend to the physical. The bodies of the people cannot be touching and should be separated by some distance so that one person's aura is not being influenced by the aura of the other person.

This has to be a lightbody experience and not a physical body experience or an aura experience. The intimacy has to be such that the individuals have a separation. It is true lightbody intimacy that is occurring in these instances. With each individual's consent, the lightbody intimacy exercises allow the participating individuals to exercise their lightbodies in intimate manners.

Indicating willingness to continue in these exercises can bring physical stimulation as well. If the people are in the same room they may hear the other person in reaction to the lightbody intimacies that occur. In controlled exercises the individuals are separated in different rooms or places.

The problems of intimacy becoming too intense might prompt the individuals to give up their exercises and become more physically intimate. The problems of intimacy are such that to be intimate on a lightbody level, the individuals must separate themselves long enough to allow their lightbodies to be intimate.

There are many forms of lightbody intimacy. In certain forms, the lightbody abilities are used to influence the other body without the other body having to do any lightbody work or exercise. These lightbody intimacy exercises were invented thousands of years ago and involve various forms of interplay, interchange, and intimacy.

The intimacy that these lightbodies are capable of depends on their training, their mastery of lightbody intimacy techniques, and the consciousness of the individuals. The individual intimacies are only achievable to certain levels depending on the consciousness of the individuals involved. What that means is that intimacy to a great degree is possible. Intimacy of a much greater, higher, or what one might term spiritual degree is possible for those who have attained those realizations.

In this entire exploration of intimacy and lightbody intimacy, one has to see that the intimacy extends not just to the physical. It extends through the intellectual, the emotional, and the spiritual.

All of these lightbodies have their intimate connections to each other through the intimacy exercises. These will connect the individual lightbodies. Individuals doing these exercises have connection to each other through their lightbodies.

One of the first lightbody exercises to attempt, for instance, is for an individual to send their lightbody to have intimate relations with another individual.

Start with individual A's lightbody lying down in their physical body. Individual B would have their lightbody leave his or her physical body and go to the physical body of individual A. They are then intimate with that person on a lightbody to physical-lightbody level. The interactions occur on and around the physical body of individual A.

What is occurring is that the mind of the individual B is in conjunction with their lightbody. Then they transfer it to the position adjoining individual A and has intimate relations with the physical body and lightbody of individual A. Individual A may have feelings on their skin or aura. The individual A's lightbody remains in their physical body, but has relations. Individual A's lightbody may extend out from their physical body in order to interact with the individual B's lightbody.

In the alternate exercise, individual A sends their lightbody to individual B and has intimate relations just outside their physical

120

body. This is lightbody to physical body-lightbody contact. These primary exercises allow the individual lightbody apprentices to actually have their lightbodies share physical to lightbody experience, interplay, and exchange.

The next types of lightbody exchange involve lightbodies meeting in various places. In the previous exercise the lightbody for one individual went to and was in the presence adjoining the physical body of the other individual. The lightbody of one participant remained within their physical body. In that case, the two lightbodies are together, but around only one physical body.

Another type of intimacy is when the lightbody of an individual actually enters the physical body of another individual. It conjoins in space in that physical body and can poke around and play around with that physical body.

At that time it is possible to have multiple lightbodies within one physical body. It is within these circumstances that there can be an intense form of intimacy. If the lightbodies achieve a certain synchronicity, harmonious balancing, and inner connectivity, then greater lightbody intimacies can occur.

If the master's lightbody enters the apprentice's physical body face on then the orientation will be in reverse. This is sometimes a rather uncomfortable experience for the apprentice when the master enters their physical body at a different angle than their lightbody's orientation. If the master turns to the same orientation of the physical body of the apprentice, then the lightbodies are able to harmonize and synchronize to particular frequencies depending on their actual resonant harmonies.

Intimacies between lightbodies depend on their resonant frequencies. It is not always possible for individuals to have harmony in their lightbodies because they may not be the exact same frequency. We all have different frequencies. Some of us harmonize better with others. Some lightbodies harmonize better with others. Our human consciousness also has harmonic resonances.

This exercise of having two lightbodies in one physical body can be very intimate and very connecting. Within it there is a possibility of attaining true harmony. It is a very strange feeling for the individual apprentice. It feels as if one has two sets of organs and everything like that. It is a big mess inside. To feel all of that, to feel the lightbody organs of the master within the apprentice is a very strange experience indeed.

In these exercises the participants may achieve a great degree of physical pleasure when in connection with one physical body. If the physical body is asleep, that is another matter. In most cases, it is better not to let the physical body fall sleep in these lightbody intimacy exercises. Full consciousness is necessary for the enjoyment of these intimate experiences.

Lightbody experiences may involve both lightbodies leaving their physical bodies and having a tryst in a place in space and time. That is a preferable type of lightbody intimacy for some. Travel to different places allows different experiences in very blissful realms. Lightbody love and intimacy is such that it allows people and their spirits to have intimacies on levels that are not normally known. These intimacies extend from the inner mind to the outer limits.

The connectivity between individuals becomes much more heightened through these intimacy exercises. Lightbody intimacy involves the connectivity between the lightbodies and activates the chakras, nadis, auric fields, and shields. There is an activation energy that increases the pleasure in the participants.

The individuals participating in these intimacy exercises are encouraged to have certain types of connectivity. This connectivity is especially heightened between a male and a female lightbody. There is a particular channeling possible between these bodies. They have an ability to have intimacies that extend throughout all of the lightbody and connect the lightbody nadis or energy channels between the male and female lightbodies. The energies they exchange on various levels can become increasingly intense. The intensity may become so great that the individuals lose themselves in their intimacy, love, and pleasure.

The full beauty of these lightbody exercises is that for individuals seeking intimacy it can bring greater and greater intimacy as the participants learn this play or foreplay. It is easy to do, so individuals that are not inclined to have physical sex may experiment with these lightbody intimacies. There will be emotional connectivity. Other endearing emotional connections could be made. This is not a light thing to take on. It is a very serious matter. Casual lightbody sex should be avoided.

Lightbody intimacy involves the connectivity that many would call true love or true intimacy. It is what individuals seek in their harmony, in their marriages, or in their relationships when they desire to be truly close to the other. How truly close to the other can you be? If you are just together physically that can only last so long and then one has to go to work or do something else. When you are in lightbody harmony you are always in a resonance with an intimate one, your love. The intimacy can extend throughout your life. If there is commitment then there can be commitment through time. This can extend throughout many lives. Lightbody intimacy is actually a way of forming relationships that may last for lifetimes.

In choosing intimate partners one has to learn how to connect lightbody and know how to disconnect lightbody if there is the necessity. Disconnecting lightbody is difficult for those who do not know how to do it. The lightbody master can show the apprentice how to sever any unwanted connections, or as many as they can, through techniques that allow lightbody separation.

Lightbody separation is a very serious matter too. It may involve counseling for emotional upsets. There may be holes in each other's auras and lightbodies where the connectivity was before. If there was not a clean separation between lightbodies, it becomes very messy and requires lightbody surgery to heal the individuals. In the quest for intimacy, one has to know how to back out of these relationships, or find a loving way to distance oneself from the other if the relationship is not harmonious.

In some cases this becomes impossible if the individuals are not strong enough or do not have the ability to sever connections. They may already be too close to each other in a relationship or a lifelong commitment. In those cases there is a difficulty and it may have to actually be lived through, but there must be certain improvements, which involve training and knowledge. This involves raising consciousness and becoming more intimate in ways that were not possible before. There are ways to elevate relationships that are not that great. For people just learning lightbody intimacy, there is the necessity to learn the tricks of getting out of problem relationships. One should at least know techniques for terminating unwanted lightbody relationships.

In getting intimate with one's mate, or one's lover, or one's sexual exercise partner, the intimacy exercises require coordination of the body. The participants may be at different locations. The lightbodies in these sets of exercises will conjoin in a particular location. The directions of the masters must be explicit enough for the participants to know exactly what they need to do in these lightbody exercises.

In most cases, an apprentice learns these exercises from a master or masters. It is best that mated masters teach apprentice couples how to have intimate lightbody love, lightbody sex, and all the lightbody intimacies that involve non-physical interaction.

These intimacies can be learned together in a classroom. Each apprentice couple can then go home alone and later become lightbody intimate together. In these lightbody exercises the apprentices need to know how to harmonize their lightbody frequencies with each other, how to enter a sacred space together, and to have what is called sacred sex, or lightbody sex.

What is the Lineage?

The lineage is composed of many people of many cultures of various genetic backgrounds. It is a basic trait that we might consider genetic. It is a psychic marker that may have physical characteristics. How can one tell if a person is within the lineage?

The characteristics of lineage are seen in the psychic signature of those individuals having lineage background blood. In examination of what is lineage, we first note that lineage is family, which is a genetic connection. Tribes have genetic and other connections. The lineage is a backwards-extending connection with parents, grandparents, and other relatives. The entire lineage structure is dependent upon relationships. The lineage is a conglomeration or affiliation of spirits, which form the path of genetic furtherance or continuation and spirit continuation. There is soul continuation through body, mind, and language when individuals are born into lineage families.

The lineage markers belong to the blood types that are passed through lineage. Blood contact is the primary method of lineage transference, i.e., through the blood of the mother, or by having interchange of blood through regular contact between men and women. Children might also have exchange of blood someway, possibly through accidents. Political considerations and treaties might stipulate that the winners agree to their affiliation through blood, which was a common practice around the world. It allows its lineage members to extend themselves in other realms. Lineages can be combined. Very sacred blood merging ceremonies and rites are performed during a lineage merging. It involves the preservation or the continuance of lineage lines through time.

What that means is that the availability of lineage intelligence to individuals within the lineage becomes possible. Those individuals that are connected to the lineage through blood are also able to contact the wisdom. The wisdom is part of the Ilokano lineage. Each lineage has certain traits that allow them to survive or has helped them survive through time. These traits are usually survival traits and cultural traits that have enhanced them.

In time, language and other intellectual pursuits contributed to the lineage characteristics. The attributes of these characteristics in individuals become prominent when the lineage is able to influence the education of young lineage members. Those that are born into the lineage are within a family of the lineage. Each lineage has its own wisdom and its own purpose that it has decided upon. The particular lineage of pursuing the psychic and the psychic surgeon abilities is one that extends back for over four thousand years. The use of these abilities by lineage members was developed thousands of years ago as well.

Practitioners of these skills are only using part of their skills. They have much greater talents. They can reach great pinnacles of awareness. They can become virtual healers of the masses if they were fully trained in their abilities. Others can learn these abilities, but it is a difficult process. It involves difficult study, training, and discipline. A real desire to have these kinds of talents in the first place has to be present before the student or the teacher pursues this adventure and training. The training itself is actually good for the student and the teacher. It furthers the connectivity of all involved with the purpose of changing the entire world through this healing process.

As a healing process, we might call this a lifelong pursuit. This is not a skill that one can learn and unlearn. Once one starts learning it, it becomes easier. It takes more and more of one's time, mind, and energy as one becomes more and more aware of the universe. One becomes aware of one's place in it and one's ability to influence the universe through one's endeavors. One becomes aware of how to coordinate with others, especially in the raising of family, the building of community, and the furtherance of the lineage through time and space. Part of our heritage is to be joined in the heritage of others.

126

Network of Life

The psychic surgeon is part of a network of life. In that network there is a certain affinity to all others. Some call it the web of life. There are many names for it. Being part of that web of life, the psychic surgeon is able to travel across it, to other places in that web, on the web, and even outside the web. The psychic surgeon's duty is to maintain the health and life within the family, clan, lineage, neighboring clans, and communities. The psychic surgeon is in tune with all that is going on.

The living vibration, the earthly vibration, the air, the stars, and everything everywhere, affects the psychic surgeon at all times. The psychic surgeon does not have to be aware of everything. Awareness is part of what makes them effective tools for God as they follow their chosen destiny. As the psychic surgeon becomes an instrument of Divine Will, there are more opportunities to use these higher God-given gifts.

I will now continue to talk about the psychic surgeon, but only use the term surgeon. The surgeon is also available for emergency operations. They pull the necessary conscious and unconscious energies together in a way that can effect healing. The healer, another term for the psychic surgeon, is aware of what is the basic default pattern of biology connected with the entity to be healed. This is usually an innate understanding that comes through a sensing of the patient. They can sense if the patient is a person, animal, insect, or another form.

The healer-surgeon is part of many worlds that other physicians would not deem necessary to be in. The role of the psychic physician is to heal, in a broad sense, by being part of the whole. Being part of the whole means using all of the whole in the healing technique. The whole or the totality is within the individual physician. The psychic physician manifests their talent in the healing situation they are in, using the totality. They may not need actual physical tools such as scalpels or other medical devices to do this surgery.

Being a psychic physician is a responsibility that extends beyond removing malignant tumors or such. It is having the ability to maintain health. The maintenance of health, the birth of life, and death are all part of the physician's duty and responsibility. It is a universal skill among those who have these kinds of talents ingrained in them. Lineages and families that have close connections care for the health of each other.

This is instinctual. It is a psychic instinct. The psychic physician uses their instincts because they know much more than they think. Much of this information is beyond the comprehension of the practitioner of psychic surgery. The psychic physician is actually a much higher discipline. It involves the entire network of healing and is not particularly emergency disease related. It is more health and life related. It involves the whole process of connectivity through family, clan, and lineage.

What this means is that genetic structure is a primary contributing factor to the overall health of the community. The actual cultural practices become ingrained in the healthy family, healthy community, healthy tribe, and healthy lineage. The tradition that is born or built up through these activities becomes the ongoing activity of the lineage one is part of.

The actual lineage of these psychic physicians has an understanding built in. They can effect healing because of their close connection to the universe and their use of tools that connect them to the universe. These tools are within them. They are simple equations possessing power that allows the individual practitioner to rise above the normal laws of space and time. They are using those laws in the manipulation of particularly isolated zones. The radius of the fingers, around the fingers, and the hand, normally determines these zones if the hand is used as the instrument of the surgeon.

Having an understanding of the complexity of relationships is essential. They can be between the individuals within the family, clan, lineage, tribe, and ultra-tribal connections to other tribes. It becomes part of the conscious awareness of what the people in the lineage talk about. These are actual relationships and language is a good vehicle for talking about these relationships. The relationships exist in an observable form to the psychic physician.

There is the necessity of maintaining the resonant harmony within the family clan and tribal groups. By being in touch with that reality, the emotional-mental problems that might be evident in a non-monitored society are actually filtered and dealt with directly through the traditions in the lineages. The actual use of this total method of comprehending relationships means that the physician can detect when things are wrong.

Physical problems, emotional problems, and mental problems are not part of the harmonic. They are not part of the resonance. These things might be diseases. They might be psychotic problems or emotional problems that could be sorted out. A physical problem might be cured through psychic surgery. The mental or emotional problems might be resolved through counseling with lineage and family members.

The availability of opportunity to progress and get over difficulties is well-inherent in the structure of tribal societies. These are what we might call the primitive family and tribal units. The connectivity between these people becomes one of health because everyone is so interconnected. It takes time from everybody's time for people to be cared for. In the overall flow of time it is realized that the prevention of disease is more effective, energy wise, than the curing of it.

The actual traditions within the tribe, society, or lineage are such that they dictate that health become a primary factor. The structure of the lineage is such that to progress there has to be love, procreation, family units, clan units, tribe units, and other broader scope relationships with other tribes or lineages within

129

the vicinity. The lineage that has psychic surgeons or psychic physicians is connected to the spiritworld, the world of nature, the earth, the sky, and the universe.

What we have in the lineage is a broader understanding that allows the individual to see the spirit in another. The psychic physician is not only treating the body. It is a matter of seeing the body and treating the spirit. The body and the spirit are healed.

Why is this? The body is more than atoms and molecules. It is composed of a lightbody, an aura, other forms that maintain its structure, its identity, and its place in space and time. The ability of the psychic surgeon depends on penetrating and altering those realities within a certain space-time network, framework, and location coordinate.

Normally this is done with the assistance of guides or other lineage members. They can help with these operations, especially if the individual performing them is not particularly schooled in this methodology. The reliance on faith and other spirits to help in the healing process is essential for the lineage practitioners. It is not the lineage's responsibility to perform miracles themselves. It is to be the instrument of those miraculous occurrences.

The humble nature of lineage members, in most cases, leads to their closeness with God, their spiritual nature, and their deeply religious convictions and devotion. Taking those considerations to heart, one can see how in time the grace in which the lineage exists can be shared in other communities and the world at large.

In understanding the entire compassionate nature of the physicians in the lineage, the idea of sharing this compassion and healing with others is part of an awareness. Lineage members are aware that we are all part of the whole. We are all whole together and we all have purpose together. When one boat rises, all boats rise.

Who is the Psychic Surgeon?

The psychic surgeon tradition is best known through its representation in the Philippines. There are other practitioners in the world that use similar or possibly the same technology. Identifying other actual practitioners of psychic surgery is especially difficult. Some may be concealing themselves from the public.

In these days the practitioners are often using their abilities in commercial practice and in an unrecognized manner. Unrecognized by science and modern medicine. It is necessary to identify the psychic surgeon to determine the authenticity of the practitioner and the efficacy or actual outcome of their healing efforts.

Their healing efforts can extend to many realms. We will start with the physical. The actual pictures, photographs, videotapes, and other visual evidence might characterize the identification of physical healing through the method of psychic surgery. There may be a growing body of actual medical evidence of why this phenomenon occurs or can occur. The entire understanding of this science, art, or practice is becoming more important. If it is indeed real, it offers an alternative to painful medical procedures and chemical medicines that have greater side effects.

Determining the actual effectiveness of these psychic surgery procedures will allow other practitioners to duplicate the methodology. The procedure and actual healing can be spread to other trained professionals. These novice surgeons can become proficient depending on their aptitude and pre-aptitude. Their predisposition to this ability is through culture, relationship, and bloodline. We find something that is possibly unique in the Ilokano lineage. Their bloodline allows them to do psychic surgical operations.

It is through bloodline that the Ilokano lineage has their ability to use psychic surgery, as it is termed, to manifest healing. These skills are best explained by mechanisms that are not explainable by known science. It is possible to explain these and that is what I will attempt to do.

For instance, the relief that the person receives from the treatment can measure the actual manifestation of the psychic healer's ability in healing another person. Being the patient of a psychic surgeon involves being part of the procedure. These procedures are often unique to the practitioner because of the lack of centralized facilities and procedural methodologies that are necessary for establishing recognized medical practices. The procedures must be documented. The documentation of these procedures must occur in a logical manner that is understandable to the layman and to the medical scientist as well.

In choosing a middle path in explanation, one would require a great deal of graphical information to make it possible for anybody interested to understand what is going on. In preparation of these graphics it is necessary to remember that we can usually represent what is going on in either a two-dimensional or three-dimensional format. The dimension of time can be seen as well.

We will speak of and define these energies in the procedural manipulation to procure healing. Procuring the psychic healing involves using energy. That means using one's ability to manipulate and manifest energy in means that are intentional. They are based on the decision of the practitioner, the will of the person needing the treatment, and the desires of their family. A practitioner may need to perform surgeries or other operations if a person is injured.

Continuing, who is the psychic surgeon? In reference to the lineage, the psychic surgeon is part of a tradition that extends back thousands of years, approximately two thousand BC for the Philippines and other places in India before that. The tradition is carried out through the family and the bloodline.

It is an oral tradition through training by family members, from elders to youngsters. Those who grow older retain the knowledge. They are the grandmothers and the grandfathers.

The spirits of deceased grandmothers and grandfathers have this knowledge. All of those in the lineage are connected and their knowledge is all connected through space and time. Each person within the lineage has a connection to others within the lineage. This connectivity goes throughout those with the bloodline in the lineage. This connectivity allows those within the lineage to use their innate abilities to perform the psychic surgery.

The surgeries are dependent upon the ability of the psychic surgeon to do manipulations that are not ordinarily used by medical surgeons. They do not have to involve surgical tools except the use of the hands. Other surgical tools are sometimes employed or have been employed.

The learning of this is usually intuitive. One sees it and one does it. Oftentimes the training occurs spontaneously and instantaneously. Those that have this ability have it within them and they know it. Knowing that may give them courage. It is not easy to do. Because of its nature, it is highly charged. It is a procedure that involves the surgeon as much as the patient. The surgeon needs to call upon and build the instruments within themselves to do the surgery.

This is accomplished through various methodologies employed by individuals who have been trained or self-trained in the procedures of psychic surgery. These procedures involve the use of one's body to influence someone else's body.

A psychic surgeon must have control over his or her own physical makeup, energies, space, and time to manipulate these energies. The psychic surgeon must transcend boundaries to accomplish certain procedures, which we would call healings. The person that is being treated is also in that area. The patient has to go into another space and time as well so that the diseased organ or afflicted area can be healed.

This is transference of the body in space and time to accomplish various purposes. These things observed in psychic surgery, such as the penetration of skin, the removal of diseased organs and objects might be characterized as miracles or unexplainable. Looking at the amount of hoaxing that can occur and how easily the famous Randi portrays it as a hoax, the actual use of these techniques to perform operations to achieve healings may be hoaxes in some cases.

In some cases these events are real. It is that realistic aspect that we will investigate. Using these particularly special innate talents makes the psychic surgeon a special person. They have an ability to heal. As all doctors know, they have an obligation for the health of others that need and want their help.

You will find that individuals who practice psychic surgery have deep faith and belief. They love humanity, the world, and animals. They love the spiritworld because they work in the spiritworld to accomplish these miracles. These may not be miracles and these may not be hoaxes either. We might characterize these occurrences as miracles because of the good they can do for the people receiving the treatments.

In our first characterization of these as miracles, we want to know if there is something that the person achieves. Using methodologies such as the classification of miracles in the Catholic Church and other religions gives us a baseline for determining if a medical procedure is indeed a miracle. If these are miracles, then why are there not more saints being canonized in the Philippines and other places where these surgeries are occurring?

The psychic surgeons may be doing miracles because they are built for it. The type of blood or other characteristics they have makes them predisposed to do this work. This work is not the calling of the entire lineage. It is the calling of those who are actually called to do it through the need and through the love.

The need is there. Within a community and family, there is often danger. People get hurt from time to time. Even on a daily basis there is danger and disease. In the spirit of caring for one's family, the people are able to share this healing. It is done in a caring way. There is an exchange that is familial, tribal, and within other interchanges with other tribal groups. Neighboring tribal groups might need the healing abilities of these people.

We call them psychic surgeons. Some have called them shamans. This is a phenomenon that extends back thousands of years. We can call it ancient, but is it something within the scope of shamanism? It is possible that we do not actually have a clear picture of these techniques, the people that practice them, and what is going on in overview.

Taking an overview perspective, we see individuals are being called to fulfill their place within their family and tribal network. If they have ability, they are awakened to use that ability. The religion that the person employs or is using at the time does not determine the outcome. A person could have any number of religions, yet be related in the lineage.

For instance, lineage members can be Christian, Muslim, Hindu, Jewish, or of any number of the other religions within their realm, grasp, and understanding. They could still use these techniques to do their healing, magic, or miracles. This phenomenon might be seen as a lineage that has a power to heal.

There are lineages everywhere and everyone has lineages. Because you are alive, they have been successful. They have produced you and your family. Hopefully you can help and produce children and a family. People around the world can help out through procreation and the furthering of their own lineages.

Finding the abilities within your lineage means that you can carry out the scope of your genetic programming. The genetic programming is more than skin deep. It goes through space and time, through your family and ancestors of so long ago. It goes through all the relationships that occurred in all the time that came to be before you were made. Now that you are, you are in a network of reality within this world, and other worlds as well.

In analyzing why a person would be interested in becoming a psychic surgeon, one starts within oneself. A person might ask, "What is my relationship to a psychic surgeon who has their own tradition, their own lineage, and their own paths? How does this relate to the knowledge I want to have, the path in life I want, the joy I want in my heart? How can I share that in my life?"

What do we see in looking at the whole scope of psychic surgery in the Philippines? The number of practitioners is growing. The knowledge is growing through sharing of books and videos.

All this is leading to a growing understanding within the world that something special is happening. It is not known what that is exactly. Understand that the psychic surgeon originally had their purpose within their own family group. This group was special to them. Their love held them together, especially among those who were more intimately related such as couples, children, mothers, fathers, grandmothers, and grandfathers.

We find that in early times the love between family members was so close and binding because so much time was spent together. Families shared a similar spirit and joy together. This is because of the paradise that these people lived in for many thousands of years. They lived in harmony with nature and the spirits there.

Sharing the world as they did allowed them to grow in peace and harmony. They cultivated abilities that were becoming more widely available as the bloodline of the people grew through interchange, intermingling, and marriages. In their wars they had peace and blood treaties. These allowed this lineage blood to be passed on to a great number of people, not just relatives.

The important factor is that a particular type of blood, not necessarily the blood type, is necessary to allow these people to do this particular healing. Taking this overview to start with, we see that these skills are not available to people without this type of blood or this blood signature. If they are, it takes extreme patience, concentration, and training to overcome the limitations that people in the lineage do not seem to have.

The important factor in all of this is not that they have any snobbish view of you. These people are humble, close to the world, nature, animals, and spirits. Looking for the psychic surgeon within these lineages, one can find it within them all, because they all have this ability. They may not know it, but it is something they could find if they were to meditate or activate it.

The activation of these people on a molecular level, genetic level, and a personal level through their minds, emotions, psyches, and spirits, allows them to influence others in a more positive manner. The awakening of psychic surgeons is very special within a community of these people. There is an understanding that if some start to understand then more start to understand. It is a mirroring of experience through time.

The more the people grow, the more they grow together and the more they grow forever. Being people within families, family groups, and lineage allows the entire culture to progress through time in harmony with their own destiny and the destiny of their group. This group is particularly dedicated to the healing process, the spiritual process, and the self-improvement process. They have so much that they do. All of these contributing factors gave the people in the lineage abilities to focus their forces on the techniques that are necessary to effect the psychic healing. They did not have to have any particular religion in the past. They were able and are still able to choose whatever religious path they wish such as Christianity, Buddhism, Islam, the Hindu religion, animism, or other more native or indigenous religions.

The understanding of the techniques from any particular religion is not necessary for the actual implementation of the psychic surgical operations. These are entirely dependent upon those within the lineage and their identity within the lineage.

Extra abilities may be attained through other training programs. For instance, the use of the Christian catechism, prayer, the sharing of religious experiences, and the worshiping of God or other deities are examples that might influence these people and their lineage. This enables them to contact the spiritworld.

Spiritworld communication is an essential ability of lineage practitioners. The contact is with the spirit and body of the person, animal, or spirit they are treating. The ability of the surgeon to transcend their own time during psychic surgical manipulations means that they are giving faith through time. The patient is going through a self-help mechanism, although it is the psychic surgeon who is actually putting their hands within, or using some other mechanism or manipulation to effect this healing.

The psychic surgical manipulation is one in which both the patient and the surgeon are transcending space and time together to effect a miracle. These miracles are within the grasp of the psychic surgeon because they are trained within. Within them there is a mechanism to provide understanding of these psychic surgical operations.

The understanding of the operation itself is entirely intuitive when the psychic surgeon becomes operational. The intuitive part of this is the actual sensing, seeing, or perceiving of the disease. The patient's problems become evident during the extension of the surgeon's lightbody into the patient. This occurs allowing the psychic surgeon to do this surgery or to do the pre-diagnosis of the patient with the special help of their lightbody abilities. Other instruments are available to those within the lineage and those using lineage tools.

The use of these tools is one that the psychic surgeon has at their grasp because it is inborn. Inborn tools are the easiest to use because the lineage has pre-programmed them for use. The tools need to be activated. The users need to be shown how to use them in particular manners. The tools are used in the healing techniques, the psychic surgery techniques, and the enlightening techniques. In the higher forms, the enlightening techniques are capable for use in psychic surgical procedures and technologies.

These technologies are available to those that have the particular blood signature. There is no guarantee that they will have any ability or success in effecting these miraculous occurrences.

As much as any individual not within the lineage would wish to teach or train, their ability with the other students is limited. They either attain this through blood or have some connection to it through lineage. Their own line may have had a trace connection with and or an installation of the tools of lineage members, that effect the transformation, miraculous healings, and other phenomenon associated with psychic healing.

This is a pattern that develops. The person developing these psychic abilities has a particular unfoldment of abilities. These are identifiable by certain stages of consciousness and their relationship to the training, to the teacher, and to the overall structure of the knowledge. Those that are going these ways or taking this path in becoming psychic surgeons are challenged by the ordinary steps those taking this journey face. These might for most include discipline, doing schedules of mediations, and using hand energies. This requires a discipline of self, patience, a desire to become much more, and to do much more for oneself and those you intend to help and heal.

The abilities of the psychic surgeon are such that the surgeon needs to have more control over their lives than most. They must be especially conscious of their time and space, protective of their environment, and particularly secretive about what they are trying to do. They are not influenced by others who might say that they are not accomplishing as much as they should, or they are on a wrong time schedule, or have no knowledge.

The dangers in any path are inherent in the path of the psychic surgeon. Learning this technology is not one that involves super-human powers. It is the same old drudgery as in any path that leads to ability. It is a talent that could be used to help others and help oneself.

The manifestation of the psychic talent in the individual might have to come through various processes. These include an ability to meditate in any particular manner for any particular time. That means to meditate either with oneself or in an envi-

139

ronment with others. It includes meditating in a team, a team of several, or a team of two. They must meditate to accomplish feats together and accomplish what is called psychic acrobatics. The ability to work together on many levels, especially the psychic, the spiritual, and the astral level, allows the teacher and the student to accomplish what they need to.

Eventually the person doing this would either be alone or with their family in the practices that are common to this lineage. The practice of this tradition can be adapted to one's lifestyle. Doing things in a particular manner enhances the ability of the psychic surgeon to do and become more than what they were.

On the path to being oneself and being a psychic surgeon, one finds that there are choices to make. These choices allow one to go farther faster and are part of the process. There are actual shortcut signs along the way. These might say meditate five more minutes a day to cut off this many weeks of your training in meditation, or something like that. There are little shortcut paths and scenic routes that people like to take along the way. These little shortcuts help people to find their way to enlightenment, use their abilities, and to use their psychic surgical abilities to facilitate the healing of others and the world.

The abilities that are innate within the psychic surgeon from this lineage give them protection. They hold an auric manifestation that allows them an ability to maneuver through the world. They hold a harmony that is not observable in most other individuals. Those in the lineage hold an ability to be bright and quick. This is identifiable in their person, what they look like, their stamina and such. This is a general characteristic.

One might observe the way they use the world, their clothing, and their things. Their connectivity with the world is somewhat different. It is appreciative, yet it is not possessive or obsessive. The lineage has an ability to embrace reality and love it for what it is. This is a benefit. The understanding within the lineage is shared from a young age to an old age. The knowledge, language, tradition, and culture are communicated and not forgotten.

The shared home, environment, and family togetherness is a building block of this experience. This makes the psychic surgeon and fulfills them in their role as a person in a family, clan, lineage, and nation. People have this inner connectivity, one to the other, not necessarily through blood, but through their relationships and understanding.

This is the path of love and sharing of love through the family, and of joy that occurs through life and birth. Other manifestations of love are through romance, sex, and procreation. On the path is the work we all do, the work done to become, to be together as families, as clans, and as a lineage. These relations extend out for many miles, for many minds, in many spaces, in many times.

The people that are within the lineage have a connection to each other through space and time. They accomplish what they can and wish in their own places. The eyes of each are within the eyes of all. The minds of each are connected to the minds of all.

The lineage is actually a part of a ring or a web that extends through wherever the consciousness will take them. Being part of the lineage is being part of the world that they are in. Being a psychic surgeon is being a person that can effect a change for the good within their family and community.

The calling of a psychic surgeon makes a person want to do more than what is just survival based. Part of survival would require that individuals within the family and tribal network have the ability to heal. This ability is inbred in the body. It is close within the psyche growing up. They have this ability to share and to propagate within space and time within their family group. They are able to share this talent and to procreate and carry on their tradition. It is important to fulfill the necessary family obligations and obligations to each within one's family. It means that one takes on life and does one's best as an individual. One does one's best to help and heal.

Helping and healing, being part of the calling of those within the lineage, has become so much a part of their work that they are actually making money at it. They can do that because they are talented at using these techniques. The use of these techniques was not necessarily confined to those of the Espiritista Christian tradition. These techniques predate that tradition. The methodologies employed by the Espiritista Church are fine. They involve the Lord Christ, God the Father Almighty, the Holy Spirit, Mother Mary, and the saints.

In reference, the idea is that the use of the path of Christianity is well within the scope of the psychic surgeon. Great faith is the tool that the psychic surgeon uses. Faith is the power that unleashes the ability. The psychic surgeon needs this faith to accomplish what is necessary in the healing process.

Using faith is the mechanism that activates the psychic surgeon's ability. The ability is there, but the faith may have to be developed. This is often done through prayer and exercises. Seeing it done effectively would convince most people, or some people. To be able to see it and do it is the turning point of the young psychic surgeon, or the novice psychic surgeon.

Effecting change within another environment is to penetrate other realities, other bodies, other beings, and to do this in a manner that is helpful. This allows those within the lineage to accomplish the goals of healing as psychic healers. The actual use of these technologies is not limited to psychic healing or psychic surgery. It is actually part of a much greater tradition that is lived in the lives of the individuals that are part of the lineage. The psychic surgeon takes a veering path towards the fulfillment of their destiny in the most natural way that they can. This is done in the most faithful and reverent manner accomplishable.

The psychic surgeon is on a path for success. This is accomplished if their heart is leading them on their path and they have great discipline and seriousness about this work. Being faithful to it is the first step. Being so disciplined that you are not going to take a misstep is very important. Being on this path to becoming a psychic surgeon means you are intending to learn more than you ever thought was imaginable or could ever imagine.

Being on the path of understanding is like a child looking at the university medical library and saying: "I want to know all this, you know." It is a vast undertaking and a vast thing to know. To become part of this entire process of relativity that psychic surgeons must accomplish is vast. They must be related not only to their family and lineage, but also to the actual patient in a way. They must have a very intimate relationship with that patient so that their hand may go in and penetrate the body and remove a tumor or do some other surgical operation.

How does one perform the healing that is done in a manner that is just right? What is necessary? What is needed? How is this accomplished? How can an uneducated surgeon accomplish all of this? How is this possible? How is that within the grasp of the psychic surgeon? Innate programming within the body of the psychic surgeon allows them to call on resources that are not available to most people. These resources are a technology that is embedded in them, allowing the psychic surgeon to do their surgical operations without incurring damage in the real world.

The use of these tools allows the psychic surgeon to manipulate their lightbody, their physical body, and the lightbody and physical body of the patient to penetrate into the patient's body and accomplish the surgical operation. The surgical operation is a part of a pattern that allows the individuals to be healed. It is something like a form of forgiveness, a form of continuance, and a form of reciprocating love within the community.

The actual healing process the psychic surgeon becomes involved with is so intense that the energy becomes magnified. The psychic surgeon may be in a different state of mind. The surgeon's physical needs must be attended to, such as warmth, water,

143

or whatever. It is a different mechanism or body pattern that they get into at that time. Self-discipline helps in maintaining the environment and the healer's own health. The problem is that a healer could try to give too much and keep giving too much, particularly if they are doing many operations per day.

The ability of the healer to do these operations is like having inborn surgical tools within their hands. They have knowledge inborn within their minds. It is using what they have to do, what they must do. To use and to gain this ability is something that one might see as the birthright of all humanity. This is not necessarily so. Knowing these techniques is part of a trade secret one might say. The use of it is confined within the Ilokano lineage.

The training involved in manifesting these abilities is vast and intense. It takes training from the age of conception to birth and beyond. This is not an easy path to take. It involves telepathic training from very young ages. In many lineage traditions the training of the unborn is the most important factor in establishing connection between the lineage and the newborn. This training must begin when the child is in the womb. The mother and the father communicate with the spirit of the child.

After birth, the mother and father must continue to train the children through telepathic means. This occurs before they are able to talk. This enforces the training methods and the ability of the child to absorb greater and greater amounts of information. The child learns to fulfill their potential as an infant.

These infants can be great thinkers and great telepathic talkers. They may not always remember what they say. A mother might record and translate it all. Using an audio recorder, she can translate and record what the baby's thinking. Some record and translate the thoughts of their pets and other people, as well.

Two entities interact in this module. The interaction has attributes. The attributes of this interaction are forms of energy, presence, thought communication, and other forms. Interaction is involved with purpose. The purpose is decided upon ahead of time. In this module, the purpose is the transmission of knowledge. The communication channel is telepathic and verbal.

The resonance established between the two entities shall be known as the teacher and the student or the master and the apprentice and so forth. These relationships exist for the benefit of the continuation of knowledge. This is the inheritance of the lineage that passes it on, the school, the college, the university, or the book. The knowledge can be gained through various forms of learning, education, and training.

The initial forms of education in this module are the initial contact between the two entities. This is the unborn child and the mother. Other relationships may exist such as unborn child and father, unborn child and God, or unborn child and other beings.

This module allows for multiple forms of relationship, but only one at the time. This module only contains two entities. In this instance, these are the mother and the unborn or the newborn.

The teacher in this instance may be the newborn or the mother. The teaching may occur simultaneously and can actually be timed. Realization is part of the teaching. That allows the parents to learn, especially if they pay attention to the newborns and the children.

In the teaching process, entity-to-entity, the collaboration to produce the result is helpful to furthering the cause of what they pursue together. Such instances of the relationship are the family relationship of mother and child, father and child, child and another person, or child and a pet.

All of these learning experiences are possible through the coordination of the interplay of the mind and the experiences with each other. Although inanimate objects can be used, there are often spirits connected with them. That may make communications more or less viable.

This involves the ability to believe and have faith. Some may not remember their early training yet can still use those built-in abilities. Those with that faith are able to use this ability in these processes. Their faith in God Almighty, Jesus, Mother Mary, and the Holy Spirit allows them to use this ability. They manifest healing within the context of their lives or in the clinics they run.

Being in touch with their faith allows them to be especially connected. This connectivity to God and the Holy Spirit is the key to unlocking the miracles of which they are capable. The connectivity to the Holy Spirit allows the psychic surgeons to use themselves as conduits of the energy. They are the tools of the Holy Spirit. The Holy Ghost is in their hands during their operations. The psychic surgeon is a vehicle or an engine of the universe, of God's universe.

In accomplishing this work through the psychic surgeon, the Holy Spirit is able to fulfill God's purpose in the alleviation of suffering within the world. The Holy Spirit uses the ability to make the world a better place through this technology.

Sharing this technology is not the wrong thing to do. The necessary training is so huge, vast, and immense that those who are trying to attain this knowledge are possibly in for a surprise. It is not just a class here and there, or a ten-month immersion. It is something you become. It is you because it is life. It is a person's connectivity to the world that allows them to be the psychic surgeon.

The path of the psychic surgeon leads to intimacy with the world, harmony with the universe, and peace with oneself. The connectivity that individuals feel leads them to want to relate and use this in relationships. The characteristics of these relationships are joy and love. These are the interests of practitioners in love, in family relationships, and in their continuing lineage.

In doing the exercises that are necessary to become attuned to the use of the energy, one will become more closely affiliated. They are affiliated with the whole family and the whole community they are within, the nation, and all the spirits therein and thereout. In becoming a psychic surgeon, one is imbued with the Holy Spirit. One has their consciousness expanded. They see themselves in their place in space and time, their place in mind, their place in a body, their place where they can become what they are, who they are, and how they are. They have the intuitive feeling for all of that.

Being part of everything and within the flow allows the surgeon to manipulate the realities within their sphere of influence. They become effective movers and shakers of the worlds in which they participate. These individuals are interested in making the world a better place. They find themselves within a community or network of souls intent on the same purpose. They are individuals with high ideals. Those high ideals lead them to goals and paths that take them to wider vistas. They can see and be more than themselves. They see what they might want to be in some future time.

In this path one is not in isolation. One can choose to be in this journey with another or others in a family, in a class, or in a group that allows this to occur. A meditation group or another group that can focus in this work together can be spiritual companions in this work. They can be a team that is able to do what a psychic team can do.

This psychic teamwork involves individuals extending from their own realm into a realm of being in communion with other spirits, with other bodies, and other lives. This connectivity with the same similar purpose is orchestrated through a training master. It allows the apprentices to congregate in any time and space to take the training. It allows them to do the training, be the training, and be healers in space and time. It allows them to do this healing in a local environment, right there with the patient, or in remote healing with other forms of this process.

The process is entirely up to the individual. It is up to the individual who is on the path to realization of their psychic surgical abilities. It is something they can accept on that path at that time. In the pursuit of one's path as a psychic surgeon, one has to understand that one is only going to get so much information along the way. Frustration must not become a matter that holds one back. Knowing that one can accomplish some of these things without direct teaching is something that one might want to pursue as well.

The use of psychic surgical tools is one thing. The learning of how to use them is the other. It is the hard part. The tools themselves are codes or codework that allow the psychic surgeon to do manipulations in space and time. The formulas act in a manner that affects the physical body, the lightbody, the emotional bodies, the spiritual bodies, and the mental bodies. The psychic surgeon is manipulating the bodies being affected in the patient. The psychic surgeon is using tools, procedures, codes, and concepts.

These concepts are divided. Each is a block and within each block is a sub-block. In each of those are procedures that go with it. There are general procedures within the procedure that one is going to accomplish. Each of the steps within a procedure is within the general framework of the knowledgebase. The knowledgebase is divided within the operations that the psychic surgeon is going to accomplish within any instance.

The accomplishment of an intrusion of hands into the body to extract diseased tissue is accomplished by taking the part of the code involving penetration and using it in the hands. Using that code in the hands means using and activating that code within the hands. It is activated in that space, in that movement, into the other space.

What is being accomplished is the activation of a particular equation. This is applied upon the physical body in real time, in physical space, to accomplish something. The other accomplishment is the knowledge of the ability to effect the healing. That is itself a self-healing. Self-healing mechanisms are accomplished by setting block organisms within the block of the body. The code is set within the afflicted area of the patient's body.

A mechanism for the genetic memory of the organ can be restored. The restoration process is memorized within the sensing organ. The code is transferred through the hands. The hands do auric and lightbody manipulations to accomplish the effect of healing. This occurs through the non-conscious or non-mental state using general desire, faith, hope, and prayer. At that time the faith, hope, and prayer help accomplish the insertion of the hand within the patient's body.

Faith and hope are at a very high degree or must be at a very high degree to accomplish this. To accomplish the penetration and the other energy manipulations requires great patience. The manipulation of natural spiritual energy is not easy. This is best accomplished if there are others helping that are within a similar frame of mind. They can be praying and sending energy up at that time. This can occur within the area and proximity of those doing the healing. A prayerful mindset is required. The sanctity of these exercises or procedures allows one to accomplish more than the physical healing.

This is accomplished by the presence of other divine spiritual entities such as Mother Mary, icons and pictures of Her, and the accomplishment of a spiritual awakening within those that are near. Considering that these techniques are not religious based, they can be used by any faith, such as the Hindu, or other faiths.

The psychic surgeon uses the ability to actually manipulate the body of the other person. This is dependent on knowledge of the flow and the actual tubing of the energies within the body. It is not necessary that one know where the organs are. One has an innate feeling of what is right and wrong within that organ.

The use of faith is especially important. The ability of the psychic healer to transcend normal means of faith and go into a miracle mode allows them to do miracles.

The psychic surgery methodology involves the manipulation of forces and fields within the body. The body of the surgeon must attune to the body of the patient. This is done through a format of consciousness. There is attunement with the consciousness of the body to present the body as a field or different force than is in the normal reality. What is occurring is that the psychic surgeon is manipulating the fields within their hand to change the environment of the hand. It is changed and enters into a realm or another dimension that the psychic surgery can be performed in.

This is a manipulation of space and time. It is a manipulation of body fields. The body field of the psychic surgeon is primary. Its effect on the patient is secondary. The patient normally receives a change because of what is going on. The actual space-time of the body of the patient is changed so that this may occur.

The energy involved is very high. There is the necessity of transcending normal boundaries of space and time. It is good for the practitioner of psychic surgery to develop high powers of concentration, prayer, and dedication to the work. Then the practitioner can muster the forces necessary to do this work. The energy comes through the psychic surgeon. The energy may be made available by the prayers and best wishes of people in a room nearby.

All these are part of the supplementary augmentation of the surgery through the intervention of energies through prayers and lying on of hands. This is accomplished by sending energy to the practitioner through prayers, or through hands that may be extended from several feet or across the room to the surgeon.

The energy manifestation necessary to transcend the boundaries is quite high. It is available to the practitioner. The practitioner of the psychic surgery has to use the energy in a form or set of procedures that allow the healing to occur.

In the practice itself, the individual is trying to use the good energy to do well. To do well is built into the methodology, so the healing part of it is a necessary part. It is not that one can learn this to do ill. This is a healing process. Using it otherwise is a different format than the healing format used by the psychic surgeons and psychic physicians.

The ability of the psychic surgeon depends on their ability to control the flows within their own body. The flows are from the hands. This is the most common tool that the psychic surgeon would use in going around the body, over the body, and penetrating it when necessary to relieve the body of stresses that are diseases. Problems might be cured, helped, or healed through the psychic surgery process.

Where is the mind of the psychic surgeon when performing this? The consciousness or the thinking part of the mind has to be focused on the details of what is going on. There has to be a procedure, knowledge, and foreknowledge of what is to be done and how one is going to do it. This is built into the process of psychic surgery. One knows or feels what is wrong. One knows or feels what needs to be done and what is true to do.

It is a natural process to do psychic surgery. The healing evolves from the harmony that has to be present in health. The connection that the healer makes with the patient is one of connectivity to harmony. It establishes a resonance within the patient's body to the harmony of the world. In the process of using psychic surgery for healing, the psychic surgeon is not just contacting chakras, or energy centers. They may be using the energy centers in their own body, in their own hand, to do this. The patient's body may not have chakras in those locations that are diseased. If they did they might not be functioning properly.

The job of the psychic physician is to maintain the healthy energy within the community. This means that the energy flow within the chakra systems of the people living in the lineage must be in harmony. The psychic physician has to be in harmony with this whole flow. The psychic physician has to extend this harmony to the individual they are relating to.

Without understanding it, individuals are able to perform this psychic surgery and to accomplish what we might call miracles. Why is this so? It is because they have faith to do this. This faith is derivable from many sources. It is faith in God and in the Holy

Spirit. In Christian forms it is faith in Jesus, Mother Mary, the Almighty, and many of the popes and saints.

All these factors might contribute to where the energy and faith is coming from to do this healing. The communion of the other teachers is essential in the healing process. In the healing process, the healer, or the psychic surgeon calls upon the knowledge of those beyond time, those connected through the lineage in the psychic healing tradition.

The people that are part of this tradition have access to entire libraries of experience. They can see through the eyes of lineage holders of bodies throughout space and time. Places that have had lineage experience are accessible. The eyes of the lineage can see where other lineage members have been.

This knowledge becomes available to those able to access it. This is through their time portal and consciousness, whether it is in this lifetime, a past lifetime, a future lifetime, through their eyes, or through the eyes of others in which they share a networking consciousness. The psychic surgeon's education may be close to no education, but they can still function as a surgeon.

The traditions in which the psychic surgeon exists and operate are actually very old. It is not like this is an upstart religion or a new cult. This is a practice that is widespread across the galaxy. The use of these procedures and techniques are so effective that they are used frequently and have a widespread use and application. The use of the psychic surgery is only a small part of the potential of these techniques.

Understanding the universal connectivity between individuals, the psychic surgeon and the patient, allows the psychic surgeon to extend their hands into the sphere of the other individual, the patient. One might see that the hand is a matrix of energy lines in this procedure if looking through the eyes of a psychic surgeon. These energy lines extend out from the chakra centers that are located at places on the hand and across the body.

Being interconnected, these centers of energy are connected by a neuro and psychic network. This allows the psychic surgeon to sense the environment through their chakras, through their body, and be aware of the environs or the universe near them. It is an extra step in an awareness of the environment. This is an awareness of the spirit and spirits in the environment. This allows psychic surgeons to harmonize themselves within the environment and harmonize the patient with a healing process.

There are reasons for having special locations for the healings. Some environments are especially conducive to healing and have been blessed. Psychic surgeons have located power conduit areas that have emanations due to magnetic lines of force. Other types of energy may emanate from particular places.

In the use of the forces, energies and fields that are available to the psychic surgeon through their hands, the psychic surgeon effects changes in the patient's aura. This can be done through intention or through the use of cooperation with spirit guides. Some spirit guides are within the lineage and trained within these techniques. There are many lineages and many techniques. We are only going to be exploring some of these that are used by the psychic surgeons of the Ilokano lineage in the Philippines.

The use of the aura or the sensing of the aura by the psychic surgeon is one of the first things to do. This can occur from a distance. The psychic surgeon does not have to be in the proximity of the patient to observe, scan, and take information regarding the individual.

In the psychic surgery process, the psychic surgeon is able to gather information before meeting the patient. The psychic surgeon can effect some pre-surgical relief either of pain or anxiety. They can have a resonance set up, so actual care is being sent and received ahead of time.

These kinds of things can be pre-set up by the psychic surgeon. To work with the other angels or people connected with the patient allows the healing process to begin. The surgeon is aware either through verbal communication or telepathic contact. There is a connection of the psychic surgeon to the environment. It allows the surgeon to take from the environment the energy necessary to effect the change within the individual. This brings out the healing.

These are not miracles that can happen all the time. One cannot put a head back on somebody who has lost his or her head! This is a life surgery. This is not a miraculous event surgery.

Even though these kinds of medicinal or surgical procedures are regarded as miracles by many religions, they should not be considered as defying the laws of science or medicine. It is just a different tool or format. It is not that this has been invented yesterday. The psychic physician, use of psychic surgery, and all of the lightbody tools have been around for thousands of years.

These tools are used elsewhere by other intelligent entities in other planetary systems all across the galaxy. We did not create these tools as humans. This is a borrowed technology. The use of this technology is not as understandable as one might hope.

In becoming a psychic surgeon one must be able to take a lot for granted. That means knowing that you are not going to know unless you are highly initiated. There are very few people that have a big enough head to absorb all that. It is more like one would need a brain the size of a whale. The brain would literally have to be the size of a whale because the knowledge is so vast.

The procedures that are used by the psychic surgeon are understandable. They are uniquely suited for a consciousness that is limited, which our human consciousness is. The limits of our space and time environment as we exist in it allow us to have certain manipulations of that space and time. The more we are able to do that the greater responsibilities go with that. Greater challenges and greater adventures go with that as well.

In this path, the psychic surgeon is not only doing well for the world, but also doing well for him or herself. He or she is having a good time at it hopefully. Rewards and happiness can be brought to all those involved. The patient, their families, and the tribal communities are strengthened by health, life and birth. In some cases the healing can continue through death and rebirth.

In this proud tradition of time and lineages, all people find themselves becoming reborn or being connected. They see their grandfathers and grandmothers in their grandchildren's eyes. The idea of transferring through time is acceptable in many cultures. We see references to this kind of thinking in the Bible. What the psychic surgeon is able to do is to see the person's place in space and time, and their destiny within their family and clan.

The surgeon sees how the person fits into their lineage. They see how that person is interconnected. They can see if that person is connected to the wrong people or energies. Those connections are examined.

In many ways these psychic surgeons not only deal with removing disease or healing within the body. They can work on removing connections that are unnecessary and unwanted. Some of these are psychic cords and strings, or psychic chains that attach individuals that should not be attached. People become attached through time, through careless relationships, through good or bad intentions, and through unavoidable and avoidable circumstances. Being a psychic surgeon also involves feeling whether individuals should cut off sources that are draining of energy, if necessary. If a psychic surgeon finds a psychic leech on a person, it should be removed.

Evil people might put energy drain connections and cords on other people. Spirits might hang around a person. There are all types of invasive spirits and cords and beings in this world. The psychic surgeons have to help in removing them and allow the person to connect with their true connections. In many cases the true connections are choked off by the unreal or the unwanted. However, they are very real. Connecting with true connections such as family connections allows the individual to re-grow those cords to their true family, to their true love.

These kinds of true connections may need to be rebuilt in individuals. That involves exercise. The psychic surgeon is able to apply this in the manipulation of the fields and cords they encounter in the patient, on the patient, around the patient, and through the patient. The psychic surgeon encounters all kinds of fields, forces, and cords when they encounter the other individual.

If one were looking at an individual through a psychic sense, one would see them with their body as only a partial shell. Out of their chakras are tubes circling around running this way and that way. Energy fields are magnificent pulsations. It is a truly beautiful thing to see the human in their true magnificence with their chakra radiance and to see the energy fields and the lines of forces connect that one individual.

It is even more amazing to see two individuals in their contact together. In their contact in various positions, the kinds of energy fields seen are made available through 3-D mind's eye spatial recreations. The intimacy involved in the psychic surgeon's ability allows them not only to perform the surgeries necessary, but also to live their life more fully. They may live their life in a more intimate manner with their mate, their family, tribe, and community because they are so connected.

Being connected gives the psychic surgeons the special talent for working within their own close-knit family, community, and tribe. Some do this on a much greater scale with strangers that are not marked with the types of blood and affinities that tribes in close proximity gain through intermarriage and closeness.

When the psychic surgeon in a non-lineage context is learning, they have a much greater challenge. They do not have the framework of family, community, and lineage that are built-in to the psychic surgeons that live in the Philippines and elsewhere. Traditions, families, and communities can be developed. The entire idea of having a healthy family and healthy community is all part of psychic surgery. In being a psychic physician one encounters not just the problems in sickness and death, but also the problems in birth and life.

The entire process of being a psychic surgeon today would involve being much more than a general practitioner or physician. It would be as a spiritual counselor as well. This is a total life position. It is highly respected and respectable. The work that is required is much greater than most. It becomes an endeavor or pursuit that requires a dedication not only of one person in the family. It is not just sending a kid off to college to become a doctor. The whole family goes. The whole family is the physician, the psychic physician. The tradition stretches on. The clan stretches on. The lineage stretches on. The tradition is within the whole family and clan. The idea that the psychic physician is an individual is one thing. The psychic physician is connected to the entire network. They are so connected that they are allowed to have connectivity through space and time and use this connective energy in their healing.

This training is more challenging for those that do not have that lineage. The people that do not have that lineage either gain connection through intermarriage or other means. They must go through a process of initiation into the mysteries of this technology. The technology itself can be transferred. It requires a special patience. It almost requires a super dedication through study, physical attunement, and exercises. It is a life-long pursuit. It allows the individual to go to greater heights. It is a family pursuit or a family matter. The individual is able to, either through circumstances or their own desires, pursue as much as they can or wish.

There is a connection between necessity and ability of local practitioners of lightbody magic. Lightbody magic is a combination of skills. These skills determine the whole fulfillment of the lightbody being, character, situations, events, and attitudes.

Lightbody magic is a procedure. As in any other procedure, lightbody magic has a certain risk. The risk in lightbody magic is that the individual participant may become too consumed by it. They could be destroyed as an individual and could not continue.

Lightbody magic employs the being as the performer, the magician, and the whole being. The individual is empowered through the magical being that they are. The being that they are and the magic that they are is inherent. They are magical by being who they are. Being present on earth is reason enough to be grateful for a position in the higher magical hierarchy.

Whether one realizes it or not, one is in a position of recognition. This is due to the vibration that emanates from the being. The being is totally immersed in the universe and the universe is totally immersed in the being. The individual is able to feel, to be the individual in the individual, and to be the individual in the whole. The individual is able to feel more and more, and be more and more. As the individual extends more, the individual is able to extend more inwardly.

As the apprentice lifts their ideals towards greater achievement, they have arms stretched to heaven and high aspirations to guide them to their loftiest goals. Others might be lead astray.

Healing with lightbody energy involves the ability to discern auric energies and auric temperatures on the body. This is done by using the perception of the third eye into the body. The presence of malignant or other diseased tissues is identifiable by the presence of unintended or discordant energies. These are easily identifiable by a soft, a yellow, or a discordant energy. These are somehow dying or are not part of the regular biological system. They may have a grayish, brownish, or another dull color. The feeling in them is difficult to ascertain because it is dead or dying. There is not much information to be gained from it. It lacks of information that is good or useful, unless one is interested in those things.

To remove unhealthy tissue from a healthy being takes the conscious awareness of the psychic surgeon. The psychic surgical being is required to do the masterly work to heal the patient.

In healing the patient there is a manifestation of a miracle on a small or great level as one might expect. The higher forms of psychic healing, lightbody healing, or lightbody surgery are not practiced because of their complexity. The complexity involved in psychic surgery involves a concentration that is unheard of in most forms of yoga or meditation. The mind of the master must be fully focused and aware of the situation to perform adequately.

In the application of psychic surgery at a distance near or far, it is important to keep track of the body, mindset, and physical reactions of the patient. In the beginning it is imperative that the feeling or the sensitivity of the healer or the lightbody worker is in harmony with the work to be done.

By feeling into the future to see events and consequences of field manipulations, the master can anticipate and correct events and problems before they occur. This is the main procedure. The entire procedure requires an alternate individual or second individual to lend assistance. A second surgeon can lend assistance immediately if the first practitioner is not able to mend a wound or do the complete healing because of complications. This is why a standby in these situations is required.

The individual giving the healing must have a mindset that is comparable with what is about to occur. If the individual is a faith healer, then the healing only has to be within the context of the individual's own belief network or belief context. It can be a simple belief in icons, Christianity, or other things that lend a power to their own innate ability. These icons are experiential motifs or media that are exploited by the individual practitioner of lightbody magic.

Lightbody magic extends into many of the magical realms on the lightbody level. These things might be adequately termed as Voodoo. Religious traditions such as the Tibetan, Japanese, and nearly all of the traditional religions employ lightbody magic. The study of lightbody magic goes back for thousands of years.

It is part of the human tradition to be lightbody beings. Some have forgotten or ignored that.

The lightbody is something that we must take into account nowadays because of its importance to the future of everyone. The important fact is that each and every individual has a lightbody. The importance of that lightbody is that it makes the future available to each individual in a much more empowering way. We are not just a physical body. We are a lightbody too. Lightbody empowerment is activation.

The lightbody activation is a means of activating the lightbody into the physical body. During the lightbody activation into the physical body, the consciousness of both becomes united and the resonance causes bliss. The resonance of bliss within the individual causes a realization of their true potential. They can possibly contact higher sources of being, faith, knowledge, and wisdom. This resonance is eternal and empowering to individual beings, groups, cultures, clans, tribes, and nations.

In our own pursuit as humans, we see our own way to fulfill our destiny. We see that our own lightbody empowers us. It is an extension of ourselves. It is what we are when we are our best. It is what we can do when we are the best that we can be. The best we have to do is the destiny of our best intentions and the destiny of God. As we fulfill our destiny we know that we are doing God's will.

Tools of the Psychic Surgeon

The psychic surgeon creates the healing tools by their use of will. The manifestation of these tools in the lightrealm allows the psychic surgeon to perform psychic surgery. Since the surgery occurs in the lightworld, the actual tools used are light tools. Using light tools is a part of becoming a psychic surgeon.

Light tools are like other tools. They have different shapes, attributes, sizes, names, characteristics, colors, and uses as well. Knowledge of these tools is essential. The knowledge of what to do with these tools is essential for those who do not have the intuitive touch that is part of the heritage of some healers. This healing touch is often passed down through the blood lineage. It usually is passed from parent to child, mother to daughter or son, father to son or daughter. It may be learned through contact with other blood relatives.

These tools do not have to be known or seen by the psychic surgeon. The psychic surgeon does not need the ability to see within the patient or have the visionary sight of lightbody sight. The talents necessary for psychic surgery are a different skill set than the lightbody teaching in totality. The total technology is one involving the teaching, understanding, and ability to cultivate these abilities.

There are certain individuals who naturally have these abilities. With little training or with training through their culture they have attained the ability to use lightbody-healing talents in their work in their communities. This is not always the case with people that do not have this heritage. They do not have this inborn training. They are not part of the heritage tradition of the lineage that has this ability. They must learn this.

The knowledge of these tools can be transmitted from the master to the apprentice through a mental process. A telepathic implantation process involves the implantation of the knowledge of all these things. The knowledgebase is so complex, diverse, out of the imagination, and beyond comprehension of the normal user that it can only be transmitted as a certain code matrix of equations.

Those relationships therein give the healer or the psychic surgeon the ability to do certain things in certain realms. These inborn tools or these acquired tools are part of the code that is activated upon need.

The activation sequence is helped through training and knowledge of what to do in the instances where psychic healing needs to occur. An intuitive feeling may enhance the ability of the psychic surgeon to detect various maladies or diseases that are treatable through this technology.

The psychic healing technology is one that involves use of interdimensional portals. These allow the psychic tools to do their work. Learning the psychic tools through training is one that involves time and telepathic communication.

The whole training is telepathically based. The use of these abilities and the lightbody technology implies the use of telepathic technology. Part of this entire process is to learn to telepathically transmit, communicate, and to do many of these tasks.

The psychic surgeon is one who learns to call upon energies that are characterized by spirits, teachers, and by masters that give this training. There has to be a knowledge transmission that occurs over time. It is part of the lineage teaching, the teaching of doctors, surgeons, healers, faith healers, psychic surgeons, and doctors of faith.

Psychic healing is something that occurs in the lightworld, lightbodyworld, or spiritworld. It implies that there can be much assistance from those beings we might call disincarnates, angels, or other beings. These beings are often part of the lineage traditions. The lineage is of the fathers, grandfathers, mothers and grandmothers. They extend back in time before these families and clans and tribes. They extend throughout regions. They extend throughout time.

The training or the experience available to the psychic surgeon is from the entire lineage. It is through that lineage that the abilities of the surgeon are activated or allowed to become possible. It is through contacting this lineage and being part of it, and being part of this training, that the faith healers can do much of their work.

Without that connection it would take the precise knowledge of what is possible. How does one do this psychic surgery using the will and imaginative abilities of a healer and surgeon? This is a matter of great training and discipline using the imaginative and cognitive abilities of the psychic surgeon. The ability has to be one in which the psychic surgeon is able to sense the malady or disease in the physical person. They must effect changes in the psychic realm, in the lightbody realm. It is with this understanding that the psychic surgeon is able to change the reality.

This changing of reality takes training that is beyond normal means. The faith healer in the traditional Filipino manner might use their ability and not know or feel what is going on. What is going is that there are many hands at work. There are many spirits at work. There are many forces at play. This surgery is very intricate. It involves a great deal of energy. It is energy that is shared across the realms. It is shared between the healer, the patient, and the spiritworld.

The portal that is opened up between places within the body of the patient is the place of a miracle. The miracle is a time portal. The time portal allows the experience and knowledge of the past psychic surgeons to gather. They share and help to do their work. They guide the energy of the physical person. The physical psychic surgeon places their hand upon and within the body of the patient and effects the change and may remove tumorous bodies or do changes within.

163

These are part of the changes in reality that occur in the other reality and can change the health of the person. This beneficial effect is accomplished through the great faith, hope, and prayers of those involved. It takes great hope and faith to effect these changes. It takes the belief that the participants can be filled with the Holy Spirit.

These are miracles of spirit and miracles of space and time. These things that happen must be attributable to God. In the prayers that proceed and follow these miraculous events, many previous lightbeings may be mentioned, called, or seen.

These beings may be from the religious past of the participants. Known lightbeings have appeared in previous miraculous happenings in the religious experience of the participants of faiths, whether they are Christian, Muslim, Jewish, Buddhist, Hindu, or any of the other religions that have had great visionaries. They have seen these lightbody phenomena manifest miracles in people's lives.

Believing in lightbody is something that usually occurs after one experiences lightbody. Lightbody experiences are sometimes simply discarded, ignored, or relegated to a dream type of world and not paid attention to. Lightbody is a real place and it is a real world. It is a place in which one can do things in an alternate reality.

It is a second life beyond normal life. It is a dimension beyond the third or fourth dimension. It is a place in space, time, and mind where things can be done that transcend normal reality. That is the reason why people choose to attempt to learn lightbody, lightbody technology, and lightbody techniques. It is like learning another skill, an athletic skill, a mental skill, or a professional skill.

Lightbody skill is another skill. It is a very hard skill to learn because it involves much of the person's life. The lightbody apprentice has to go into oneself to draw upon an inner power to become a lightbody player

164

Lightbody Physician

The lightbody physician has to determine if there is a problem and then find a specialist in lightbody technology that can perform the appropriate operation. The appropriate operation for each condition may take a number of repeat operations with various levels of recuperation. This is not an easy process. It is best left to the psychic surgeon or those who have the ability, either real world doctors or psychiatrists. They do what they do best. Lightbody technology and theory does not take the place of modern medicine except when necessary. This is characteristic of most lightbody uses. Lightbody technology is within the legal frameworks of society, within societal norms, and accepted behavior patterns. It is within the families and family groups that exhibit these powers, abilities, or senses.

These are the talents of the lightbody healers. The lightbody workers have a much greater purpose than healing. They help the whole person, not just in healing the physical body, but also by healing the whole person.

That is because lightbody workers have connection to the whole person and connection to the whole. By connecting themselves between the patient and the infinite whole, the patient is reconnected to that whole. They can gain the resonance necessary for health. In our limited existence in our physical bodies we need to resonate in health with the lightbody we have.

The lightbody is a mirror image of oneself that needs to be nurtured, protected, and sustained. That sustenance comes through our own efforts. As owners of our physical body we are also owners of our lightbody. We must pay attention to it, listen to it, listen to one's inner guide, and listen to the spiritual self within. Lightbody technology involves taking charge of oneself, of one's own lightbody, and of one's own destiny. Lightbody technology means that one can use the resources available to lightbody technicians to do certain things.

Certain talents one has and one's imaginative abilities determine these things. In using the hands, for instance, one needs to use the fingers in a manner not known to modern science. What one needs to do is to extend the lightbody beyond the fingers to distant spots. That means one has to see the lightbody extending out from the hands to those places. If one can sustain a vision of that happening, one can manifest lightbody at a distance.

Lightbody projection is part of lightbody training. Being a lightbody worker means that one works with the physical body, but the lightbody does all the hard work. As a physical person, the patients being worked on do not disturb the lightworker either psychically or physically. The lightbody worker can work at a distance or be right there with the patient.

Lightbody work is a matter of using the proximity or distance healing methods to do projective work with one's lightbody. One can project the lightbody from the physical body to distant locations and do the actual work that is envisioned. Holding the hands in the desired positions when performing the lightbody work at a certain location, either near or far, does this. With the lightbody hands in position, one makes lightbody movements depending on what one sees with the lightbody mind, eyes, intuition, and senses. Going through these motions helps the process.

As a lightbody person, one is able to tune in with the universe and also tune in with the patient, the process, the healing, and with space and time. This gives the lightbody technician an idea of what has to happen in a sequential manner. A step-by-step methodical process occurs with the lightbody worker's guidance.

In preparation for that, the lightbody worker needs to think logically, organize precisely, and have a good idea of what might happen. Because of their training they might know that certain things might veer them off path. They would have to take little distractions in stride and to come back to the focus of their work.

Lightbody Healing

Lightbody healing is like psychic healing or faith healing. It is characterized by the lightbody that is healed. The faith healing may have actual implications for the physical body and the healing thereof. The use of psychic healing or psychic surgery is a physical form manifestation. Lightbody healing is only related to the lightbody. The healings may have real implications and consequences for the physical body, the mental body, the emotional body, and other associated bodies.

The practitioner who learns these skills from the master, teacher, doctor, master psychic surgeon, faith healer, lightbody healer, or master lightbody healer can accomplish lightbody healing. All these designations of the teacher are part of many traditions. The practice is very similar. The lightbody teaching allows for use of different belief modalities. Different religions can use this lightbody healing technology.

In the preparation of the apprentice for lightbody healing, the teacher or master must have some contact with the student, be that in the physical realm or otherwise. That contact is the acknowledgement of the student and their lightbody. When the master is able to use their talents in actual service in the world, they must make contact with the student or their patient.

This lightbody technology and training is part of a major or overall training program. The overall program is a life-training program. It implies interrelationships between family members with these skills. These are clan, tribal, and lineage connections. These connections are shared throughout the region with others that are in need of certain talents, skills, or services.

The lightbody worker has to be trained in this technology. The technology itself for the most part has been an intuitive training. The practitioners intuitively know what to do. In most instances they do not feel what is happening. It is beyond the realm of their comprehension and their sensory ability to actually know what is going on and what they are affecting.

The lightbody technology training would show the student what is actually going on and how they can accomplish it with their own mind, imagination, and willpower. It takes faith and much belief in this to make it happen. That is why those participating in this should have a great amount of faith. The master, patient, doctor, and student should have faith. Faith is not necessary. Faith helps.

The faith that people have in this process or this occurrence allows a greater miracle to happen. The energy given to the situation allows the portal of space and time to be opened for the healing to occur. What is occurring is an opening of a portal in space and time where this magical occurrence of the lightbody healing can occur. It occurs in the physical realm as well.

To manifest these portals in space-time for purposes of healing, the apprentice must learn how to manipulate space-time. That implies knowing about space-time. The teacher will familiarize the student with instances of identifying various positions in space-time. This means that the student will do exercises in which they will place their mind or consciousness within various locations in space-time.

The teacher will observe this and there will be appropriate acknowledgement. This process of learning to manipulate one's consciousness in space-time is a primary requisite. It is through space-time that the lightbody can be contacted and manipulated. Space-time is a continuum. The apprentice is only opening up a small part of that continuum. It is like putting one's hand in a running stream. The stream continues, but the hand stays there and the stream goes around it.

Only if one is immersed in the stream of space-time is one able to go with that flow. In this reality, individuals who are apprentices, patients, and masters are taking their time in this time, in this continuum of space and time.

When learning about space and time, the student has to be aware of their particular and unique place in space-time. This implies responsibility. The space-time continuum allows individuals to train in space-time consciousness at a much-accelerated basis. It establishes a consciousness interchange or a communications path or tunnel between the apprentice and the teacher.

This communication allows space-time training to be accelerated beyond the imagination of the apprentice. Knowledge of space-time is such that a little bit is a lot. A lot is just a little. The more you know, the more you know you do not know. It is a continuous loop. Keeping conscious about it or knowing it logically is a difficult task for anybody, the master included. Having an overall grasp of the space-time reality is necessary for the master and the apprentice. It is not necessary for the patient.

Space-time consciousness is one that allows the master and apprentice to go through time and space portals to accomplish the healing, task, or mission at hand. Space-time is a place. It is also a time.

There are various locations, such as locations on earth, in space, on various other planets or realms, that are important as destinations and learning facilities. Space-time consciousness is one that is shared once the individual apprentice can achieve a certain level of conscious integrity or realization. They can maintain that awareness for the length of time that is necessary. They can use these abilities in any way possible.

The individual has to pursue their own level of expertise and they will be challenged by their own limitations. By pursuing a healing program, they can learn about the possibilities in space-time training. They can accomplish and learn what is not accomplishable by normal methods or normal efforts. Having a direction in the training is especially important to begin with. Lightbody healing takes the devotion of a medical scholar because of its complexity.

The teacher's task is to train the apprentice. The task of the apprentice is to learn, to know, understand, and manipulate all the energies and influences involved. This goes along with knowing the attributes of the lightbody and using these attributes or manipulating these attributes for the purpose of healing.

Having a classroom situation allows the lightbody training to occur in the real world, for acknowledgement of the teacher, other co-students, or co-teachers. Because of the nature of lightbody training, individuals will advance at their own pace. As they advance they will all eventually reach similar plateaus that the teacher or master is able to establish for that classroom or that class regime.

Lightbody training takes the form of training in the meditative disciplines. These are enhanced by the ability to concentrate for any length of time. Concentration is the key to meditation. In its purest form it does not allow deviation from the path of true concentration, attention, and focus upon the purpose.

The concentration involved is necessary for the student to attain the higher goals and realizations of this practice. The teacher has a responsibility to describe and demonstrate concentration. The student is graded on their ability to concentrate for various lengths of time such as one minute, five minutes, ten minutes, and thirty minutes.

This testing of the ability of the apprentice to concentrate is necessary. If the apprentice is going to do any lightbody work, they must be in a concentrative or meditative state for the amount of time that the work is done. It would take a half-an-hour of concentration to do a mission that was a half-an-hour mission. Having these abilities and the ability to meditate and concentrate for extended lengths of time is an asset for the lightbody worker.

The lightbody can have enhanced energy through physical health. Those using their lightbody in lightbody work are advised to stay in physical condition that is good or even excellent. Good nutrition and various forms of exercise are advised.

Lightbody Surgery

Lightbody surgery involves many forms of surgery simultaneously. The lightbody surgeon works on many levels in several dimensions. The surgeon coordinates the activities of other lightbody entities, spirits, angels, or beings known by other names.

Lightbody surgery in most cases involves multiple layers of surgical operations. The lightbody surgeon has various responsibilities. They must first determine the damage to the patient's physical body, lightbody, and auric bodies, if possible. Any other bodies that are available for consideration should be examined.

Lightbody healing occurs at various levels and times. The sequencing of lightbody healing is a matter of choice by the lightbody physician. The lightbody physician uses their lightbody mind to make a diagnosis.

Lightbody surgery in most cases will first involve working on the outer auric shells that are related to any condition that will be treated. For instance, if an arm were to be treated in a healing, the auric energy around the arm at various distances would also have to be addressed in the healing.

A congruence of factors that are applicable to lightbody surgery has to be met before lightbody surgery can begin. Under the strict conditions of beginning lightbody surgery, the lightbody surgeon must first pay strict attention to the methodology of the practice to be done. In the next few procedures the lightbody technician must have clarity of mind, spirit, and purpose. They must have clear instructions on the procedure to be done.

Lightbody manifestation in the psychic surgical procedure involves instrument holding, instrument analysis, instrument manipulation, instrument insertion, instrument removal, and instrument disposal. The procedure and procedure analysis is omitted here.

The entire structure of the procedure is based on lightbody analysis. Lightbody analysis is determined by the emissions on or from the lightbody. Making lightbody analysis by the lightbody technician or the lightbody worker is important. Making determinations about the lightbody according to certain lightbody specifications, requirements, baselines, or defaults is important. When entering the lightbody information into the conscious database it is important to know the system of analysis being used. The attitudes of the lightbody worker and patient are important.

The system of lightbody analysis has to be considered in view of the lightbody worker and the lightbody patient. There is not a good analysis until there is a firm congruence, confluence, or agreement on the aspects of the lightbody manifestation. This includes the lightbody, lightbody power, lightbody emanation or lightfield, lightbody auras, lightbody chakras, lightbody in physical body, and other energies within the body that include electrical, neurological, and reflexive energies within the body. The entire structure of this thought pattern is applicable to the physical and the kinesthetic powers of the body in its manifestation of lightbody powers.

We have the power of all within. This is the emanation of the power of the hands and the emanation of spirit. Spirit is able to manifest in the body of the healer, to be transferred to the body of the patient by applying the proximity healing technique. This means applying the body of the healer's hand within an inch or two within the proximity of the body or within the body to affect the cure. Having hands that can do what one wants is supreme.

The lightbody healer is a healer that uses their lightbody to do the healing instead of their physical body. The lightbody is available to do lightbody healing at a few inches away from the physical body, or very close to the physical body. The lightbody healer can heal from a distance or from very great distances away from the physical body of the patient.

Lightbody surgery is a matter of placing the lightbody of the lightbody surgeon in various proximity positions to the patient's physical body, auric body, or lightbody. The lightbody surgeon must be sensitive to the patient's various other bodies, besides their physical body, to treat these simultaneously.

In the coordination of lightbody treatments through the use of manipulative techniques on the physical, emotional, mental, auric, energy, and lightbody fields, the lightbody surgeon or lightbody healer intuitively feels what needs to be healed because of its lack of resonance with the universal resonance of good vibration.

It is easy for the lightbody healer to perform healings because the healings are corrective actions. These can be done instantly or over a matter of time. A few minutes are normal for some lightbody healings. Longer times may be necessary. These lightbody healings or procedures usually take as long as the lightbody healer needs to take to do them.

If they are following a procedure based on a religious practice or another practice, then they may have a prescribed path and possible rituals involved with it so that the healing can occur in a manner at a particular time, or take a certain amount of time to say certain words, think certain thoughts, or say certain prayers.

All of these accompanying activities to lightbody healing are part of the lightbody process. It is part of the lightbody education in many cultures to learn an entire body of knowledge or set of procedures in order to perform the lightbody healing described here. The lightbody healings can be classifiable by their attributes of healing the physical, emotional, intellectual, auric, and lightbody.

Lightbody healing as performed by a lightbody healer or a lightbody surgeon is a matter of synchronizing the patient with the universal vibration of wholeness. The lightbody technician is actually a person or being that can synchronize the person or patient with the whole and restore well-being. Using lightbody

173

technology to heal is part of a healing process that is shared throughout all of humanity and across the universe. It is a loving lightbody universal fellowship.

When performing lightbody healing on a patient or oneself, one may find that there are physical reactions like the involuntary reflexes that occur when a doctor hits one on the knee or other knee-jerk places.

This may occur even if the lightbody physician's body is not in proximity to the patient's physical body. There may be a physical reaction on the body of the patient and physician. This is observable in people with great auric and lightbody sensitivity. It is an attribute of one who has a more sensitive lightfield that extends out from the lightbody.

The lightfield is like the auric field except that the lightfield is much greater and much farther reaching. It is composed of various different types of vibration and is not related to the physical body itself. Lightfield is related to the lightbody. Lightfield is the aura of the lightbody. Lightbody emanations or lightbody aura can extend from a few inches to great distances, depending on the available energy source for the lightbody illumination.

Lightbody illumination is like turning on a light in a lightbody. The light expanding out of the lightbody can expand to various distances, illuminating other lightbodies in the presence of the lightbody energy that emanates from the person that is emanating lightbody energy. The availability of lightbody energy is also dependent on the individual lightbody worker's ability to tap into that energy. That energy is infinite. The ability of the lightbody worker is finite.

In finding the happy medium between the finite ability of the lightworker and the infinite amount of light energy available is a matter of learning procedures and being able to channel greater and greater amounts of light energy into the lightbody. This requires quite an amount of experience. That is gained by simply doing it over and over again. Over time, having the illuminating experience of light in the lightbody will give the lightbody worker the ability to channel even greater amounts of light.

In the process of learning to be an active lightworker, the individual has to take small steps in the activation of their lightbody. This normally requires practice. This starts out as a difficult procedure, endeavor, or hobby. It is something that can be rewarding and it has greater rewards than one might imagine.

Lightbody workers in training need to learn to concentrate and think properly. By concentrating it means to apply the attention directly to their mission. This is difficult to do for most individuals. The lightbody teacher or master will have to show the students how to attain patience and discipline. The students need to do that so they can do their lightwork.

In this lightwork, the light procedures become second nature. They allow the lightbody apprentice and master to use the energy that is available. If they have manifested a channeling experience, the energy will be flowing through them without their having to think about it. As it becomes more of a procedure of active channeling, it becomes less of a thinking procedure.

As each step of lightbody illumination unfoldment occurs, the individual lightbody master or apprentice can proceed to much greater levels. In understanding the lightbody illumination process, the lightbody worker has to be able to know where their energy is coming from and where it is going. They are aware that the lightbody energy will flow through them. They will become the conduit. The lightworker is the conduit of the lightbody energy. This lightbody energy is often called Spirit, Holy Spirit, or Spirit of God.

There are many types of energy that are available and convertible to forms of light energy. In most cases, the lightbody beings maintain their lightbodies in various energy forms and formats. There is not any particular vibration or frequency that all lightbodies have to manifest on. Lightbodies are quite inventive in choosing various frequencies for the manifestation of their lightbody energy.

Because the lightbody energy is the energy that is used in the healing process, the lightbody workers are learning to use themselves for this lightbody energy to perform the lightbody healing. The greater amount of discipline they find in themselves, the easier it becomes to do the healing. In doing this healing, most practices have deep devotional requirements and religious overtones.

The belief of the lightbody master and apprentice must be very great for these things to occur. These lightbody healings require the belief of the lightbody worker in most cases. In the beginning, the lightbody worker does not have to actually believe in order to perform their lightbody work. After they see a healing they believe.

Lightbody work is easy to do because it is all part of a natural intuitive process that everybody knows. The more that one tunes into the lightbody work, the more one can learn about it and know about it. It is all part of the process. Some have forgotten our connection to our lightbody. We have religious institutions to help us remember that connection. Lightbody workers need to be able to focus themselves and to focus the energy upon the lightbody healings they will perform in their lightwork.

Lightbody to lightbody surgery is a difficult process unless one is a lightbody master. In the healing of other lightbodies, the apprentice must first learn this process before they can practice it because of the damage that can be done by improper lightbody manipulation. As the apprentice learns various lightbody healing techniques, they can eventually become lightbody healers of other lightbodies.

In the initial lightbody healing techniques, or learning steps, the lightbody apprentice learns how to use their own lightbody to heal various levels of the patient's aura, or another's aura. In most cases this will be done by using their hands in the proximity of several inches to several feet away or even farther.

The lightbody apprentice should learn to use their hands to manifest the lightbody energy at various distances. This energy must be used in the healing process. This energy is transferable from the lightbody of the lightbody master across the distance from the master's lightbody to the aura of the patient. The apprentice must learn how to do this.

Feeling the aura, the auric levels, the auric vibrations, and the auric shells is the normal process of lightbody healing of auras. The lightbody worker will analyze the lightbody connections, auric connections, physical connections, and cords on the client. Then there is the removal of items such as implants and other unnecessary debris that can clutter up the individual. In most cases these removals have to be arranged with the individuals and it may require a session with the lightbody surgeon. Unnecessary connections are cut. The body is then attuned and healed.

The lightbody apprentice must have their act cleaned up before beginning this lightbody work. The lightbody master helps the apprentice with this. The lightbody master sees the apprentice's difficulty in this and sees the problems. The master sees what is wrong with the lightbody apprentice and helps them remove those obstacles. Those obstacles may be implants, spirits, demons that haunt, cords that tie them to people, events in the past, emotional connections, or psychological loops and barriers. Some things are not easily dealt with. The lightbody master can deal with some things by performing a lightbody healing. This healing might be quite intensive depending on the problems of the apprentice.

In the lightbody activation, the lightbody apprentice would find that they could achieve certain forms of lightbody enlightenment, but that it requires certain steps to maintain it. The lightbody master can open the apprentice's eyes for a limited amount of time so that they can see the beauty, the heights, and the majesty of what they are trying to attain. When the master no longer holds the door open for the student, the student learns to open the door. The students must learn to clean the window and all of that. It is part of the lightbody process.

The dispensation of spiritual energy into the physical body or the lightbody of an individual is not always dependent on their spirituality or their ability to receive that energy. Spiritual energy can inhabit individuals because of previous connections with spiritual energy. Other entities may inhabit the physical body of a person and give them spiritual energy of some form.

An example of this would be when a spiritual being that is emanating high spiritual energy is also cohabiting a physical body with a regular person who has a normal spiritual energy. The normal person may not have the consciousness to use higher spiritual energy. That higher spiritual energy may be due to the presence of an angel, an elevated being, an ancestor, or a being that is part of that individual's lineage.

However, high energy is not an indication of a higher spirit. It could be an intrusive spirit. It could be an invading spirit that is just out to have fun and take in the sights. The energy might be exhilarating, but it may not be a higher spiritual energy. That is the danger.

In any individual's recognition of their own lightbody, they have to recognize what is theirs and what is not theirs. They have to learn to differentiate. They may only have a small amount of energy compared to the other entity that is occupying their body with them. The person should be content with the guest beings' energy or make them leave.

The individual must be careful of making deals or arrangements with entities that visit them. The individual must beware of using another entity's energy without very good reason. The only good reasons for working with entities are spiritual reasons based on true involvements and true commitments through time. These are usually based on spiritual and love commitments. Involvements should not be allowed if they are otherwise.

The lightbody dispensation in an individual can come through one's own lightbody or through the lightbody of another entity that is cohabiting. We will start by analyzing the instance of a person who is the only inhabitant of the physical body. One who has control over one's physical body and is not being cohabited by another spirit has options to use, manipulate, or dispense the spirit energy, or the Holy Spirit energy if one has that connection.

The higher the connection the individual lightworker has with Holy Spirit energy, the more efficacious. Better effects are possible according to tradition. If making a higher connection is not possible, there are entities and spirits on lower levels that afford various types of healing. Their abilities are not as great, not as spiritual, and may have strings attached. Those kind of lower connections are unpalatable and can cause problems. Lower spirits can make the situation worse. The higher the spirit called upon, the better. Call the highest spirits to help do the lightbody work. It is better for the lightbody worker, the patient, and all involved.

The lightbody dispensation of lightbody energy in the form of spirit energy can be directed through intelligence. This is a spiritual intelligence that is made available to the lightbody worker. They connect to the spiritual intelligence network of information. That information is made available through their own intuitive resources such as their own ability to feel and understand the situation. The information is in the form of lightbody vibrations, emanations of individuals in their proximity, auric influences, and interactions. There are also physical, mental, emotional, verbal, and other interactions within the realm that the lightbody worker works.

All of these influences become part of the lightbody worker's base frame of reference. It is the chart of the patient as the lightbody worker begins their analysis and diagnosis of the situation. Then begins the dispensation of the lightbody treatment. The lightbody therapies that are provided to the patient through the lightbody dispensation can be in the form of information about homeopathic, naturopathic, or other methods of healing that would have to be verified by a scientific doctor.

There is information that becomes available to the lightbody worker when using their own intuitive skills or when using instruments such as crystals to make the work easier. The dispensation of lightbody energy through the lightbody worker is a dispensation of spirit and spiritual energy. The spirit is actually dispensing itself through the lightbody worker. This makes the lightbody worker a channel for the Holy Spirit or the high spirit that makes possible the healing.

The healing that occurs is a spiritual healing. It is a gift of the lightbody worker or the lightbody healer, yet the actual healing must be attributed to spirit or the Holy Spirit. The actual benefits to the patient are attributable to the presence of the lightbody spirit, the light Holy Spirit. The effect of being in the presence of that spirit is the desired effect for the lightbody worker. The lightbody worker establishes lightbody portals. These light portals in space and time allow the spirit energy to enter through that portal and do its work, which is the healing of the patient.

This healing reestablishes the health of the lightbody of the patient. Then it reestablishes the physical health. There may be activities that the lightbody worker may perform in doing this such as moving their hands at a distance from the patient's body in simulation of various forms of activity, such as removing of disease or bad vibrations from the body. This should be done at a distance of at least several inches to begin with as an apprentice learns to have an effect on the lightbody field. The lightbody worker will apply their skills according to the level of their skills, and the lightbody master will apply their skills as necessary.

Learning to work with spirit is part of every religion's training. Spirit is spirit. We know spirit. Some of us know spirit by different names, but we feel it in approximately the same way with different intensities.

What occurs in individuals around the world is that they have been filled with spirit by various exercises such as praying, singing, dancing, and other practices that bring about the formation of the portals of the spirit energy transference.

Opening these space-time portals is like opening a spring that keeps gushing out water. It can become a river of spirit if the lightbody worker is able to manifest that. Larger lightbody portals can be established when lightbody workers work in cooperation for lightbody energy to be transmitted. This is a function of the lightbody community of healing. Lightbody healers have an ability to do things in close proximity. This is usually because of their training, ability, and mastery of the situations in which they are involved, such as a lightbody to patient relationship. In that healing relationship the individual lightbody worker uses their lightbody to do the healing on the patient, the patient's lightbody, auric bodies, and other bodies.

In a larger context, several lightbody workers working together can accomplish different things because they have more to work with than one lightbody. They can do more complex healings that involve more parts of the patient's body being worked on at one time. Multiple lightbody workers can even work on multiple patients. There are many variations on light-workers working together. These are subjects for greater explanation later.

There are players in all of these fields of healing. They are necessary to maintain the life of the nation, or all nations, and all peoples. These people fulfill these functions in relation to everybody within their community. It is a growing experience. They are the professionals that provide training in the lightbody experience. They are the clerics of all faiths.

The lightbody worker can inspire the apprentice or patient to have visionary experiences during the lightbody work. These visionary experiences can have content from the patient's religious or cultural background. The vision may be related to the lightbody healing that is occurring or it may have another theme.

The lightbody environment that is established in the healing can influence the patient in ways that are not normal. The patient may have visionary experiences as described and other physical manifestations such as involuntary physical motion, involuntary talking or speaking in tongues, and involuntary writing. Trance-like conditions can occur spontaneously during the healing. Pre-existing medical conditions may suddenly manifest. During the lightbody healing it is advisable that lightbody technicians are available to restrain the patient or help the lightbody worker if anything goes amiss.

Lightbody work can be dangerous for some lightbody workers if they try to treat someone with a serious demon that is violent and resists the lightbody work. The lightbody worker must beware of treating those who have bad intentions. They must avoid those skeptics who do not believe. Those people might actually damage the lightbody work. This is a word of caution. The lightbody worker is in a precarious position in these times. The lightbody work is in flux and in a state of investigation. As in any new science, it will take investigation of the highest order. Research using scientific methods must be done with many case studies to verify techniques and procedures.

The cure may be real or thought to be real. The penetration may be real or thought to be real. The effect may be real or thought to be real. The entire procedure may be real or thought to be real. The manifestation may be real or thought to be real.

The judgment must be real. All skeptics have opinions that must be respected. We must make certain determinations based on the skeptic's opinions. Psychic healing, lightbody healing, lightbody magic, and lightbody are all subject to scrutiny of the imagination, of the thinking logical mind, of all scholarship, medicine, and time. Lightbody magic, lightbody medicine, and lightbody are all under attack. Lightbody is a system that is used by all indigenous cultures to heal lightbody. Lightbody is not defined by modern medical practice.

The lightbody worker does not have to prove anything or provide procedures to investigators. That lightbody work is within their lightbody culture. It is inherently part of their tradition. It is owned by their tradition. It cannot be stolen or copyrighted, but it can be copied. The ideas that are part of lightbody traditions are universal. It is common sense to know lightbody technology. We have a lightbody residing within us, or most of us do.

The lightbody understanding is part of that universal lightbody awareness. To understand lightbody work one may need to look to previous celebrated lightbody workers in one's own religion. How did they use lightbody energy to perform miracles of faith or bring people to greater understanding?

The lightbody work can be respected across religious barriers. Lightbody illumination and understanding transcends any particular faith, religion, or practice. Cultural traditions associated with lightbody enhancement or enlightenment are part of the full color and scope of the lightbody myth and tradition. This makes lightbody colorful, entertaining, and worthy of study.

In using lightbody, one needs to understand that in today's age, there may be resistance. There may be people that do not believe in using lightbody and the Holy Spirit in healing. Those people refuse to be moved by the Spirit, to be taken by the Spirit, or have anything to do with the Spirit. For some that is for good reason. They have their own faith, their own belief, and their own stability within that.

As lightbody workers in these times, we must beware of harassment and subjugation to restrictions on our ability to use our lightbody energy. We must observe the laws and norms of the societies where we practice our lightbody work, but we demand that we can practice lightbody as part of our tradition, faith, and lineage. We must be true to our faith, as our faith demands. We must practice our lightbody work in the manner that we must.

Lightbody technicians or lightworkers may have to practice privately if there is no avenue for public practice of lightbody work. The lightbody workers may be subject to harassment from the majority religion or other faiths that have antagonism, conflict, or non-belief in this technology.

Lightbody workers are not limited to having any particular religious affiliation. They can be agnostic and have no real religious beliefs. The lightbody worker does not even have to believe in what is happening. They may consider it a scientific principle of life. We can accept that. This lightbody is part of the universe. It has definable principles and attributes that will eventually be scientifically measured.

The lightbody technology has long been available to peoples around the world of all religions and faiths. Indigenous peoples had and still have shamans and their own religious traditions. Animists have a connection with this life force, this spirit force, and can use that force. Those who have respect for the animal totems have respect for lightbeings. These totems are lightbeings and have light energy, lightbodies, and can do lightbody work.

Across the spectrum of this earth's religions there is a full understanding of lightbody. Intolerance of another religion's lightbody experience causes problems. One might learn something from other lightbody practitioners if one has a universal lightbody understanding.

Universal lightbody understanding is part of the entire vibratory network that all lightbodies are connected to and are part of. Each individual person, each individual lightbody, is part of a lightbody network. They are connected to other lightbodies in their environment, their proximity, and across the world. They are connected to their family, work, and community.

There are other types of connectivity. The lightbody connectivity between individual lightbody spirits allows lightbody communication to occur over a wide network or over a wide consciousness of lightbodies. This lightbody intelligence or lightbody communication goes beyond the normal consciousness of most people. It is part of the lightbody conscious network.

The lightbody conscious network connects all individuals who have the lightbody vibration. Our human vibratory frequency connects our conscious human frequencies together. There are multitudes of variations and combinations of lightbody frequencies. Lightbody connectivity allows lightbodies to communicate.

In the consideration of the methodology of lightbody surgery, let us first explore how psychic surgery is done in the Philippines. They are using the methods of faith healers or psychic surgeons. These psychic surgeons or faith healers rely on an innate ability to effect change. This is due to the connection to their lineage. When their hands move within the body, it is actually thousands, hundreds, tens, or another number of guides and spirits that are near. They are in that portal helping that psychic surgeon doing that work.

They are all participants in this work. Some of the more skilled ones actually participate in the surgery by placing their tiny hands, miniaturized hands, lightbody hands, into the area of the portal. This is the effected area. They work together to do the great number of operations that are necessary to fulfill any psychic surgical maneuver or procedure.

The moving of the hand through the body is accomplished by placing the hand and the body in another time and space. This is possible by using the faith of the healer, the faith of the patient, or those nearby who send their prayers and well wishes towards the operation and the individual. They supply an intensity of energy that the psychic healer or the psychic surgeon is able to draw upon. This energy is focused into the area of the wound or other diseased part. Their efforts must not distract the lightworker.

The hand is the normal tool of the healer or surgeon that is used in the procedure to perform the surgery. The hand must penetrate the body of the patient and the light-time continuum. The light-time continuum that is established through this interchange determines the ripple in the space-time boundary. That ripple extends as far as is necessary when lineage members guide the actual procedure.

When the procedure is unguided or under the direction of the master, the actual moving of the hand through the body has to be very controlled. Each of the cells of the diseased patient must be totally analyzed. The entire procedure has to be one in which the psychic surgeon has an understanding of what is actually going on with the diseased part. Medical knowledge comes in handy.

The difference is that the intuitive healer would not need medical knowledge or need to see exactly what is going on. Their presence is the effecter of the change or the healing. It is through their guidance from the lineage that allows them to make the motions in the body and do the things that they are doing.

They may not know that they reach into a tumor or do something else, but that is what they do. What happens is that the hand of the healer becomes a form of container. The container of this light energy is shaped by the fingers and the cup of the hand, allowing it to shield the diseased part from the other parts. In this entire procedure the lightbody of the healer or master is actually in the body and protecting the body of the patient as well.

If this is not intuitive knowledge then it must be learned. It is a lengthy process unless one can pick it up and draw upon the intuitive knowledge of their ancestors who share the lineage knowledge. Special teachers are necessary for advanced teaching. The other way is so much harder and more difficult. It takes the brains and the time that most people would not find available. Those pursuing medical knowledge might pursue this. Some medical practitioners may want to augment their medical skills with psychic surgery. This is a methodology that would allow those that have that specific medical knowledge to do the work that they need to do.

The allowance of the individual to penetrate through various space-times is part of a meditative process that actually opens portals. The participants energize these portals in space and time. One needs to look at examples of portals in the past to know what a portal is. Portals have appeared as openings in the sky. The face of God or an angel might appear in a portal. Rectangular or circular openings, mystical caves, and magical doors have appeared as portals.

There are many types of portals. Portals to other dimensions can open up in the presence of observers. It is through these portals that entities may be seen. Observers may see a void on the other side. They may only see the mechanism of the portal itself if they do not look too far.

The activation of portals and the creation of portals is not an easy matter for most people. Most human beings are not trained in the activation of portals. The portal technology is part of this entire lightbody technology. The lightbody is a body that is in a different space and time. It is contacted, realized, or seen through the eyes of those who can see through the veils into other realities and other parts of space-time.

The easiest portal creation methodology is to establish space-time portals through the eyes. The gazers of ancient times used crystals and other mediums to see into portals. These portals of space and time allow the gazer to see where their mind will take them. In many cases the gazer was taken to other places they may not have known about or wanted to go. They might have met entities that they did not know about and maybe did not want to know.

It all developed into a great science of creating portals. These portals are places in which this healing or these miracles can occur. There are many practices throughout the world that help people make a connection with the space-time world. These allow inclined individuals to create portals through certain inclinations, religious practices, yoga, various exercises, and self-help books.

There are many avenues to take to achieve the knowledge of making portals. It is a magical tradition in itself. It is all about having access to these portals and the beings that lie on the other side. These beings can be known as lightbeings. They are pictured through history. They are quite real in that realm. They must be given their due respect and not be venerated unless they deserve one's veneration and are worthy of it.

There is danger of using the lightbody without adequate protection such as religious protection. That protection may come from devotion to God or the whole, the embodiment of God within the Trinity, the Holy Spirit, Jesus, or Mary, the Mother of God. Other religions have various aspects of God or portrayals of lightbeings that are summoned for protection.

The lightbeings in many of these methodologies are very humanlike. Some of them are monstrous to our human perception and unrealistic in regard to evidence of actual creatures or animals that lived on earth in the past. The apprentice will encounter beings with entirely different physiologies, consciousness, and purposes in this lightbody realm.

Psychic bodyguards, guardian angels, and companion spirits are all part of many cultures' knowledge, experience, legends, and lore. The whole idea of having companion spirits is part of this. Some children have companion spirits and single adults may have companion spirits that visit them. These spirits are of a nature that may be resident to a place or a person. These may even be predatory spirits. Some spirits visit people. A person should be either not vulnerable to spirits, or be able to defend themselves from them, or they may become subject to them.

The kinds of guardian spirits that accompany people in this world range from angels to other types of beings. Lightbody entities exist all around the world. These beings may have special significance to a particular culture and to those people these beings are usually known as protectorate beings because they do things to help the people that believe in them. These lightbeings are probably best described as local deities and are part of the whole lightbody phenomena. They are real, but they are of the lightbody. These beings have power over their own lightbodies. They have enough mastery of their own lightbody skills to manifest in this world to people in physical bodies.

In doing the lightbody surgery, one may encounter all kinds of energies. It is necessary to have the right types of entities in presence during the surgery. That is why much prayer is called for. People on the parameter of the operation may help with prayers. Prayers and devotion can establish the entire framework of a portal in space-time. Prayer allows the healer to draw upon the abundant ambient energy that allows healing to occur in that situation, whether it is a psychic healing clinic or elsewhere.

The ability of the two types of healers, one that relies on a lineage of healers, and the other that relies on their own technical know-how, can have the same effect and success or even failure. This is not a guarantied procedure. In any of these, psychic healing is not a remedy for death. It is a factor that may help the individual to live, grow, or heal, but it is not a substitute for God's will.

These healings are seen in the spiritworld as energetic events. As seen from the lineages of the patient it is rather shocking. It is amazing to them that their kin can be connected to the psychic realm and other realms that they are in through these portals. It is a very binding experience to perform these surgeries. It not only binds the healer with the patient temporarily, but it brings the patient's lineage spirits in closer contact.

This is necessary so that they can help effect the changes in the body of the patient. Those using these psychic surgical methods are mainly contacting spirits whether they are trained in spirits or not. To not use spirits in this energetic healing would possibly be a violation of the trust placed in the living gene and body of the person. They are all there. It is the individual at the moment that has to protect their own lineage, their own genes, and their own identity in the process of growth and life.

The psychic surgeon may encounter objects and entities within the patient that must be removed. These things may be natural or unnatural. The things that might be removed are inanimate objects and tumors. It may be a blockage that the hand of the psychic surgeon can effect a change in and the blockage is corrected. Other problems can be healed. The healing process requires a great amount of manipulation on a rather microscopic level.

It is not easy for the knowledgeable doctor to do all of this without their actual tools, scalpel, and equipment needed for an operation. They must use their knowledge, experience in visualization, psychic capability, and skills. Even though they may not have the lineage skills, they should be able to use their lightbody skills in these operations. Their lightbody has to be trained in these procedures and techniques so that it can do lightwork.

The direction of the lightbody by a scientifically coordinated consciousness is essential towards the continuation of this methodology. The methodology used by the lightbody physician is one in which they use the parts of their knowledge that are accessible. These can be images of cutting through or around diseased tissue to remove it, and using a light scalpel to do the same.

The hand is seen as the separating device, such as a scalpel. Because the hand is in another place in space and time, it can feel between the diseased and healthy tissues. It can separate those tissues by the lightfield within the emanation from their hand within the body. They separate the good from the bad as it were.

This motion within the body can be quick and rather seamless. The intuitive healer does not need to have much knowledge of anatomy. What is going on within the body is not necessarily good for the intuitive healer to know if they are not inclined to know. It is more necessary that they have faith to do what they can do to allow the entire healing process to occur.

The scientific healer or the doctor of psychic surgery has to feel and sense what the physical body requires. It requires them to have an entire knowledge of the body, the processes and placement of the organs, the energies emitted from these organs, and the usual problems encountered in the anatomy of the patient. This knowledge is learned through education and attending medical school. It is not available to the regular practitioner of psychic surgery.

The psychic surgeon is one that can take a much greater knowledgebase into this practice if they have that knowledgebase. It is eventually necessary that some psychic surgeons learn real surgery as well. There can be a complete knowledge of the procedural concept of psychic surgery. Psychic surgeons will eventually use modern technology. The most sophisticated medical equipment will be used by the psychic surgeons of the future.

The approaches to psychic surgery are varied. The psychic surgery traditions are varied. They exist mainly in the Philippines. There are psychic surgery traditions in Brazil and other places where faith healing and other forms of miraculous healing are pursued, observed, and practiced. The entire lightbody teaching has been fragmented over the centuries. In ancient times there was great knowledge about lightbody.

Lightbody technology is an inherent right of the people of the earth. It is something that can be pursued that is not dependent on a religion, social place, or profession. Lightbody is a technology. It is like learning a skill such as mathematics or physics. In this case there is the possibility of learning the lightbody healing surgical technology as well. Other lightbody technologies require advanced math and science.

The lightbody surgeon must employ a variety of tools, devices, and equipment to perform lightbody surgery, lightbody healing, lightbody massage, and lightbody. There are many categories of lightbody. Other characteristics of this lightbody healing methodology are that the physical body undergoes change. The healing techniques of lightbody surgery are best described as a healing on the physical body. The lightbody is connected to the physical body. That connection manifests in the physical healing.

The physical body of the patient undergoes healing. This change is part of the healing process. What is occurring is a complete healing of the individual. Through this healing the individual can get in contact with their lightbody and other bodies. They can then overcome the disease or problem.

In the lightbody surgery there is the factor of knowledge and enlightenment being transmitted through the healer into the patient. Lightbody surgery involves a degree of high energy. There may be high energy residue present in the individual undergoing this surgery. The amount of psychic energy required to do this work is miniscule compared to the amount of ability necessary to control the energy. The ability to control that energy is the entire key to psychic surgery.

The minuteness of every operation takes a microscopic consciousness to comprehend the detail. It is painstaking work. Healing is effected in a psychic surgical manner when working in very close proximity to the diseased portions of the physical body.

The methodology employed by physicians in the real world may be employed in the lightworld. The goal is that these lightbody techniques be perfected. Then the regular physical invasive types of surgery are not necessary as often. What we are asking is that the apprentice learn to do miracles by doing light surgery in pressing circumstances. Where light surgery is necessary and required, a light surgeon is required.

What is necessary is that those inquiring or desiring to be light surgeons need to be identified as willing to undergo this process of becoming light surgeons. Light surgery is the use of these light tools to perfect the body, protect the body, operate the body, or to operate on the body.

What we find in these operations is that the mind of the light surgeon has to go deeply into the body, into the problem, into the problem area and receive impressions. They receive visions of the exact problem that is occurring at that scale. They know exactly what the problem is without having to do anything more than to look at it.

Usually the problem is identifiable by the pain or by the patient's own expression of what the problem is. It is wise to try to discern these things by gazing into the aura, the body, and the lightbody of the being or entity, whether it is human, animal, plant, fish, rock, or a place.

All of these things have characteristics or attributes that the lightbody mechanic can adjust. Lightbody technicians can learn to become lightbody mechanics by using lightbody equipment. The lightbody mechanisms available for most mammals include auric presence, identity presence, spirit presence, and other factors. These primary factors identified are available for scrutiny by the lightbody physicians. Becoming a lightbody physician allows the person to know more about who they are by looking at more than most doctors do.

The lightbody surgeon uses their tools in this technology. These tools are usually one of their hands, the right or the left hand, or both hands in unison. Other tools are available, but some are not prescribed for lightbody surgery. The participants, who are the master or apprentice and patient, are able to perform these lightbody surgeries through the practice of lightbody procedures.

The necessity of allowing a student to learn the lightbody methodologies is part of this tradition. Even if a person does not have talent at it, they should have the availability of the knowledge. They can learn this knowledge if it ever appears in them spontaneously or naturally. The person is able to manifest capabilities of this psychic surgical technique in practice through indigenous absorption of knowledge. In their practice of psychic surgery, they have the identity of the being they are dealing with. This is the main entity that they will be addressing with their psychic senses.

They are able to adjust their consciousness, to take their consciousness and manipulate it and harmonize and resonate with the being. They can analyze, feel, see, and empathize with the being in a particular manner. This allows information to flow. This information is about the being and about whatever condition it is that needs correction. This information is available if one has guides, spirit guides, and guidance of physicians from other realms. Guidance may be about any procedure that the light physician has to perform.

Doing duty as a light doctor is necessary for many that do not perform regular medicine. Having skills in medical light doctor technology means that the individual is able to participate in the entire future of the lightbody. This is a personal health, nutrition, and consciousness expansion procedure. It is available to those who can make contact with their lightbody and use it in ways that lightbodies can be used.

The simple techniques that are presented here offer a conscious realization of lightbody capabilities. These are available to the individual. They offer the skills to perform difficult and complex surgeries. The surgeries are necessary to solve problems in the community and the family. These knowledge-based procedures are always based on empathy, sympathy, love, and devotion to one's family, neighbors, friends, clan, lineage, and other affiliated tribal groups.

It is wise to affiliate oneself and to receive and give healing and not to cause trouble or bad vibrations. We are all sensitive beings in our world. Some of us are so sensitive that we need our own turf. Maybe that is why there are so many people demanding to have things their own way. They are sensitive to everybody else wanting that too. Everybody is joining and chiming in. Because of this, there is a big ruckus on the psychic energy circuit.

We as individuals and lightbody individuals can try to protect ourselves by being psychically secure instead of psychic sponges.

The entire lightbody experience demands that lightbody people enjoy themselves in a lightbody way and in a physical way as well. This means being politically correct on many levels, not just the physical level, but on the lightbody level, spiritual level, as well as the political level. One has to take account of oneself, one's resources, who one is, and what one wants to be. Guide the lightbody and then one's lightbody will guide one through experience.

In lightbody surgery one has to learn through the experience of others. Being in contact with the teachers and souls of those who have performed psychic surgery enhances the intuitive capabilities of the psychic surgeon. One can immediately absorb those talents and abilities when necessary. This is a special skill of indigenous peoples who have had contact with their native ancestors, lineages, teachers, and their teachers' teachers as well.

What happens in this transference of knowledge is that the individual can contribute to the whole. The continuance of the race, the culture, the lineage within the families and the entire tribal group or the groups affiliated with them is achieved.

This is something that unites clans and cultures together. It is something that is built-in. It is a natural talent for humans because humans are more than their physical bodies.

Lightbody Tools

Lightbody tools are created for lightbody surgery, healing, and other procedures. Various materials are used to create these tools. Some of the materials that exist in the physical realm have physical composition. Other tools are virtual or spiritual. Those tools exist in dimensions that are beyond the physical dimension. The lightbody worker can use tools to accomplish their lightbody work. The lightbody worker uses the properties of the tool to create certain vibrations or effects.

The distance that the tool is from the work area usually limits the effects of physical tools. Other spiritual objects, such as religious artifacts, can have greater effects at greater distances. Once lightbody tools are initiated into service, they are of a different composition than the physical objects they were made from. Those tools can be used in different dimensions. There are many objects that can be fashioned for lightbody work. Minerals are used to transfer lightbody energy. Crystals are especially effective energy transfer devices. Quartz is particularly handy because of its low cost and effectiveness as a transmission device.

Other minerals and objects may be used to open portals in space-time to do the lightbody work. The lightbody tools are fashioned for the purpose of opening portals and doing lightbody magic. The lightbody worker will concentrate the tool's effects upon a specific area located within the space-time continuum. Healings, activations, enlightenments, or effects will occur there. The lightbody master guides the apprentice in the use of the tools.

Quartz crystals may be the easiest tools to begin working with. Natural quartz crystals have been used for thousands of years in this healing. These natural crystals have a natural capacity to be used to open space-time portals. Crystals have been used as space-time portals for gazing into the future or past. The use of crystals in electronic devices such as radios and televisions is well-known. The quartz crystal is capable of receiving and sending vibrations.

The apprentice is taught how to use crystals in order to know how to use actual physical materials in the real world. The lightbody master should examine the lightbody tools before the apprentice begins to use them to determine their capability to do any good. The tool must be appropriate for the apprentice to use.

Using tools that are inappropriate is dangerous. Using a tool that is too powerful is not good for the beginner apprentice. Using a tool that is meaningless in the context that it is being used is like driving in a screw with a hammer instead of a screwdriver.

It is necessary to create specifically tuned instruments to create certain space-time portals. Creating these tools and devices is the prerequisite to using them. The master should provide a working set of temporary training tools for the apprentice to work with at the beginning. Eventually the apprentices will create their own set of lightbody tools. If the apprentice has a set of lightbody tools, then the master can examine and approve them.

The original set of tools may be crystals of natural formation. Fused, laboratory grown, or reconstituted quartz crystals have qualities that are considered good for the transmission and reception of energies, influences, and information. Laboratory grown quartz is preferred because of its purity and composition. These tools can be shaped and fashioned from fused quartz. Using these tools for healing can be dramatic if there is penetration into the physical body.

Other minerals, such as obsidian, can be used. Instruments or precision devices can be created from minerals for the purpose of lightbody healing. These minerals can be more powerful if they are in their pure state and not mixed with other minerals. Using combinations of minerals is a more complex topic. Using metals is in the realm of lightbody doctors and physicians. Apprentice lightbody workers do not normally learn to use metal tools until after they have mastered the use of crystals and mineral tools.

Removing Implants

Removing psychic implants is a matter of great importance to the mission of the lightbody worker. The assigned mission may be to remove implants from certain individuals. Mission control determines who and what is done. The permission of the individual is required to remove these implants. It is like getting tires changed or getting stitches for a wound. Removing implants is the job of the psychic surgeon. The psychic surgeon can learn this quickly or it may take a while.

There are many types of implants that are classifiable as either natural or unnatural. They came with the body or they came to the body. In any case, if they are not part of what the lightbeing needs in its growth process, they are alien beings or devices. They may be classified as implants upon the physical body and the lightbody. There are consequences of not dealing with lightbody implants, psychic implants, or ET implants. They are known by other names, as well.

Implants have a characteristic of usually being invisible. This is another term for being cloaked, unseen, or mysteriously hidden. These devices are prevalent in the world. Most people that own them are being owned by them. The host is prone to ignorance and manipulation. Aliens and other intruding beings have implanted much of the human population with remote control implant devices. The problem is that many of us do not even know it.

Manipulation of whole populations is possible by using artificial or natural implant devices. These become part of the landscape, part of the psychic environment, and the world at large. They are prevalent. Any organization, association, or alliance of lightbeings with lightbodies and physical bodies wants to prevent manifestation of unwanted beings, intruding lightbodies, and alien structures such as implants.

The host of the implant is often depleted in some way. The host may have no idea about the implant. They may have no knowledge, awareness, feeling, or sense of it. The host being may not be aware of it at all. Others may notice differences in the behavior, attitude, and awareness of the host when another entity or implanted device is present. Psychic surgery is necessary to remove host implants. Implants have great influence on the decisions and destiny of the host.

Implants can be removed through detection and a removable process. The detection process is done through using one's psychic senses to ascertain if the individual has an implant. These implants are visible to the eyes of the lightbody worker. These lightbody implants are not seen in the physical world.

These lightbody implants have significance when used by other beings to control the physical body and mind of the person on earth. These implant devices are handy for beings in alternate realities and intelligences in other worlds or universes. Implants are not good for our human preservation. These devices exist in much of the population.

The implant devices exist on many dimensional levels and can be accessed and controlled by beings on those levels. Psychic implants can be biological, auric, or lightbody constructed devices that do not have a biological or material basis.

The implant may appear as a square construction in the head. The implants come in many shapes and sizes. The implant may be an advanced circuitry bypass device that bypasses the natural psychic circuitry of the mind. Those that do implants are doctors and many have the ability to rewire the mind of the host and do very malicious things.

Before having an implant removed, one would probably believe one is free and clear of such implant devices. One cannot imagine having an implant device inserted anywhere. These devices normally have no visible effect on the host's life although their mental functioning and thinking process may be compromised. People with these devices may eventually change their opinions for no good reason and become proponents of the agenda of the beings that planted the implants.

An example of this might be someone who believes in the self-determination of humanity and then changes his or her opinion and comes to believe that UFOs are here to save humanity from the right to self-determination for whatever reasons given such as to save the planet. These implant devices actually prepare the host for contact with alien life and conformity to their agendas. The implant device may make an alien life form appear to be human to the host. The host may turn a blind eye to out of the ordinary events occurring right in front of them. Implant devices also make it possible to input virtual experiences into the memory of the host victim.

Multiple host victims may share false or virtual experiences together. Implant devices allow subconscious telepathic communication between host victims. The implant device may also help to subconsciously synchronize the activities of the host victims and make it possible for them to meet by coincidence. Implant devices often gain power when in proximity to other implant devices using the same or similar technology. When enough devices are implanted in the population there is the possibility of installing herd instinct consciousness into multiple hosts creating situations where irrational opinions and behavior prevail.

People in power are most often targeted for implants. The majority opinion of entire populations can shift dramatically in a short period of time by use of these implant devices. Often an unrealistic opinion is sustained by the implants until it is no longer possible to perpetuate it. These implant devices are used by humans, aliens, and multidimensional beings as well.

Removing an implant in brain area involves removing the device, removing implant wires and connections, tubes, and other devices connecting the implant device with the host. A psychic surgeon might use the surgical tools installed in their hands and fingers to do implant removal. A lightbody surgeon might use a lightbody implant removal device.

Implant removal is a very interesting operation. It is done by a psychic surgeon in physical, spiritual, or lightbody form. The surgeon removes the bypass circuits in this operation. These circuits may be only a few or there can be millions of little connecting traces in the aura and lightbody. This is like circuitry inside the head. The implant circuitry is implanted in order to bypass the natural circuitry. The implant device makes one believe that one has control of oneself.

The device does not have to be totally operational in order to be effective. It is not used most of the time. It is only activated for testing and to take actual control of the host. The control does not have to be complete. Control of the body may manifest as unexpected physical reactions such as exhaustion or drowsiness without reason. Mental control may manifest as irrational decisions or emotional eruptions.

Implant devices downgrade the host's functioning. The implant device downgrades mental, spiritual, auric, energetic, and lightbody functioning. All these things are possible if there are implants inside the host. Implants do this because of their ability to take control of entities, physical bodies, and minds, especially of those who are weakened, in distress, hurt, injured, or have mental problems. All of these things can contribute to a person's becoming vulnerable to being taken over by malicious beings.

The psychic surgeon makes contact with the auric or lightbody traces that are connected to the implant device and removes each of the connections to the device one by one. Then the proper connections are reestablished in the brain and mind by the psychic surgeon. The mind of the patient has to be reconstructed and returned to the state it was previously, if possible. There may be localized trauma in the form of spasms and other physical reactions to the psychic surgery.

Using psychic surgery techniques on the head is more complicated than on other parts of the body. Removing implant devices from the head should only be done by master psychic surgeons. It takes a very experienced psychic surgeon to do implant removal from the head. Other organs and parts of the body are less crucial or critical. Removing implants can have a profound effect on the mental functioning of the patient and is a dangerous operation.

Malicious implant devices are often implanted a piece at a time until a complex implant device is constructed in the lightbody of the host victim. Head implant devices are usually implanted when the host is asleep or otherwise mentally incapacitated. The implant devices can be inserted little by little. The whole device does not have to be inserted at one time. The base or housing for the device might be implanted first. Then the power connections, coils and such are inserted. There are very many different device designs.

The common link between the beings on these multi-dimensional levels is that we are all lightbody beings. We live in a lightbody universe. Lightbodies have their own different agendas yet are all under the banner of lightbody.

Some lightbodies like to take human bodies and use them for life. Lightbody beings love life. The main reason the invasive lightbodies invade anywhere is to live, just like any other being that enjoys life. The experience of life is what lightbodies like to do. They do it all over the universe.

Lightbodies exist in tiny cells and large beings. Many types of lightbodies can live together in a lightbody community. You as a person are a lightbody community. You have many types of organisms within you that have their own lightbodies and they work together and contribute to make you. You must protect all of your bodies from implant devices.

Healing Codes

In the chapter titled *Lightbody Technology* there is the sentence, *"This tradition was actually began by Lord Vishnu in the translation of a particular text."* The particular text refers to the Great Hall of Records that Vishnu was translating at the time. Vishnu simplified that entire system of wisdom into a set of codes or formulas. The ayurvedic healing system used by the psychic surgeons was based on use of Vishnu's set of formulas, which was based on the arrangement of a select set of the symbols. Vishnu claims to be the creator, author, owner, and the one to go to if one wanted to learn how to use these codes the way he intended. This is a simpler grammar of the codebook formulas located on the black monoliths in the Great Hall of Records.

Vishnu crafted a shorthand version of the Hall of Records and wrote it in relief on a white stone, which became known as the Philosopher's Stone because it held the secret to transformation or transmutation. The characters were raised above the surface of the tablets. They symbolize universal concepts of math and science. This may be the lapis code that has the power of transformation. Other stones attain power with this code. There may still be copies of the code written on flat stones or on cylinders in ancient ruins. These glyphs are similar to the stylized *CARET* glyphs and can be field activated for real world use when used in diagrams and geometric patterns. The energy and power created depends on the material or device they are imprinted on.

The Hall of Records near the Great Pyramid in Egypt uses the same type of writing that is used in the lapis code found on the white stone. The Great Hall of Records might be considered as the model for the concept of the Philosopher's Stone, but it is a set of monolithic stones devoted to various disciplines. The symbols are raised in relief. The monoliths are black until they are read and then the characters being read are illuminated. Any one of these monoliths is in itself a Philosopher's Stone, but the information is presented in a generalized format that explains how things are and not how to make them into what you want them to be and do what you want, which is an attribute of magic.

The Great Hall of Records is a library and is primarily a system of documenting the concepts of physics, math, and science using symbols or characters that have significance when interpreted alone. These characters can also be combined with other characters to form character concepts in the topic being viewed.

The amount of information in this library is beyond human comprehension. It can only be investigated in small sections that have relevance. The Great Hall of Records has many galleries maintained by the ancient ones. It appears to be made of a smooth black metallic or stone material. Many viewers can view the same sections of the monoliths and see only what they are learning, because the monoliths can coordinate with the viewers and present the desired concepts in terms of logical equations and multidimensional graphical representations. This Hall of Records is a copy of many similar libraries located in various parts of this galaxy where these symbols are commonly recognized, used, and adapted for use in various localities by beings with various forms.

This library is not the akashic records, which are much more comprehensive and contain personal information about a person's past, present, and future lives or incarnations.

Finding a stone that converts lead to gold or water to wine or an old person into a young person might be done with forms of chemistry in the future. If the Philosopher's Stone is actually a tool for transformation, then there may be a multitude of uses that would entice more than the greedy, intoxicated, elderly, and the poor to seek it. These codes are built into the physical and spiritual bodies of some people. Those without these codes built-in have to learn or obtain them. Some people have the symbols of the Philosopher's Stone inscribed within their genes through the code arrangement of their genetic material. This makes it possible for some natural faith healers to heal naturally because the healing codes are inherited. Some genetic lines have weaker code images or lightbody forms of their codes. These codes images can be retraced and rebuilt through lightbody recollection and recovery techniques using meditation and other disciplines.

The codebook formulas are essentially a user's guide to the complete library. The sequence of letters is essentially a sequence of equations that apply to multidimensional situations. This is the language of that great knowledge. That is why it gains its popularity, as it is applicable to lightbodies of lightbeings across the universe. Those who have access to that code knowledge have access to the great knowledge in the universe. Beings such as so-called demigods and others also know this knowledge. These beings are very real and very creative. The earth may not be their first home. They may visit here occasionally.

The codes can be used in various manners. Copies of the entire manuscript can be miniaturized and located on the fingertips, palm, or other parts of the body. This is the preferred method as the surgeon has access to the complete library of codes and will naturally use the most appropriate codes necessary for the operations. Spirit helpers also have access to the complete library of codes and would choose the most appropriate tool necessary for any particular part of the procedure.

Segments of the manuscript or code sets can be miniaturized and located on the fingertips, palm, or other parts of the body. Using segments of the entire manuscript allows the surgeon to use the more specific capabilities of the tool set. This method is preferred for surgeons that have medical knowledge and can direct the code tools in their specific applications.

Because of the vast array of code sets available, the surgeon should learn about the methodologies of manipulating various code types, tools, procedures, or environmental factors. Using code sets limits the scope of the surgeon's task, but by itself is not a holistic approach to health.

The codes may also be used for personal protection. Codes can be placed at different parts of a person's body for protection. A single character code can be effective for establishing a particular effect. Alphabet letters are often used as single character codes. Special signs, glyphs, and sigils are also used. Multiple character codes are effective for more complicated tasks such as filtering out certain vibrations or emitting vibrations at various frequencies and timings. Geometric patterns have multiple uses.

The codes may be the magic trick that allows some practitioners to use apparently therapeutic sleight-of-hand techniques to induce the so-called placebo healings and cures. In some cases the slight-of-hand surgeon might imitate bare-hands surgery and then display various items or even blood and organs to engender belief in the power of the healing. Placebo-healing effects are not intended to substitute for actual surgery. These built-in codes allow the dramatic and dynamic intervention into the body to affect the bare-hands psychic surgery. The activated codes are used in conjunction with the Holy Spirit energy that is transferred through the surgeon to the patient.

Using other code sets can be effective within the context of the particular system they are in and the language used. An ancient Egyptian hieroglyphic inscription might be useful for some applications, but its use and procedure for use might be different than from a Vishnu code. Different codes in different scripts or languages can be used for the same effect.

In considering the codebook formulas and their arrangement in the limited application that they address, it is possible to take the same concepts and apply them to other sciences. The translation to Vedic principles is probably the easiest. The framework structure seen in the codebook formulas is a gateway to great knowledge. Reducing these essential abbreviations from the main library into thought form equation sets allows the user to address certain issues that are not necessarily part of the greater set, but are specialized towards particular applications.

The Ambassador Crystal

This chapter is about an experience I, Lance Carter, had with a special quartz crystal. At a party, my friend Charles Grotsky asked me to meditate with a quartz crystal that he bought at a fair. There were all kinds of big and fancy colorful crystals, but the lady in the crystal booth said, "This little crystal is calling out to you." I was shown the little crystal. It had a little base attached with wax only. Inside it appeared to have about seven perfect pyramids stacked one on top of another with spaces in between each pyramid. Crystal expert DaEl Walker told Charles that he had never seen a crystal like it before!

Charles said that many people told him that it was a very powerful crystal and that it was a generator crystal. I took it and started to hold it for a minute. Charles said a lot of people had held it before and had felt great energy coming from it.

Then Charles said, "If anybody can tell me what is going on with this crystal, it's you Lance." So I sat there and tried to communicate with the crystal. I held it in my hands and after a few minutes I got a connection with the crystal and got a connection with the consciousness in the crystal. The consciousness was not very interested in me. It was as if I was just another person holding the crystal and meditating on it and maybe trying to pull some energy out of it or put energy in it or force energy through it or any number of things like that. The crystal was sort of ambivalent and had the attitude that, "You are just another one of those flesh and blood beings touching the crystal."

The crystal had a little pointed top so I put it on the table beside me and meditated with it for a while. I found that the spirit was sort of evasive. When I finally contacted the being it seemed to be really intelligent and telepathic and had a lot of power. It had a lot more power than any crystal that I had actually touched and come in contact with.

The interesting thing is that when I first initiated psychic contact with it, my whole body shook, sort of a jolt, an electric shock of some nature. That passed after a moment so I kept trying to contact the spirit in the crystal, but it seemed to be going around in circles not wanting to communicate with me too much.

I could tell that it had a consciousness that extended from itself into the entire mineral kingdom out beyond its own little crystal. It was connected. That crystal was very different. I had worked with crystals and crystal balls since elementary school and had gazed into them and contacted the spirits in the crystals and told fortunes by scrying into crystals. I had not come into contact with a being with such power and force. This crystal seemed well-adjusted, but seemed annoyed that a human would try to communicate with it. It seemed to be saying, "You are just another puny human being. I'll just swim around in my crystal."

I started to try to feel what the crystal was, but that it was not only connected to the entire matrix of the earth, but also to the mineral kingdom. There was a type of consciousness that stretched beyond this crystal itself and inhabited the core of our world and other crystal places. It was not just confined to quartz crystals or other crystals. It was not confined at all.

I asked, "Are you confined to this crystal?" It was an absurd question to the crystal consciousness. It turned out that the being inhabited the crystal for that crystal's properties, its purity and its ability to be a transmitter because of its actual structure. Knowing that quartz crystals are used for tuning radios and other frequency related equipment and scientific purposes, I understood that wow, this crystal is actually inhabited by an intelligent being.

Then I wondered, is this life or is this just intelligence inhabiting a particular time and space? Why did it inhabit that crystal? It inhabited that crystal as a home because it was a perfect crystal or nearly perfect. I felt that when I contacted the entity in the crystal that there was some minor impurity in the middle of the crystal, kind of a void, and that was the place where that spirit lived or focused itself. I am not sure if it was at that point all the time. So I concentrated on that point and tried to ask it "What is it that you do?" It did not have an answer. "What do you mean?" it replied as if it was not a valid question. The crystal had an air of superiority about it as if I could not know or fathom all of this because it is so complicated. When I started to probe the consciousness of this crystal being, I started to see structures of crystalline matrices and especially felt and saw energy patterns in a matrix during the visualization that occurred when I was thinking about the crystal and trying to communicate with it.

This meditation went on for approximately ten minutes and during that time I felt a number of contacts with the crystal and some of those were stronger. Some of those contacts caused my body to shake a little by a jolt and my mind opened a lot. I was sort of transported into this crystalline realm all of those times and into the intelligence that seemed to be a vast intelligence - one not confined to this particular crystal. Its aura stretched around for a long ways.

Then I said to myself, maybe this is as far as I should go right now. This is not my crystal. I could feel its power, but I could not use that power. It was a power unto itself. It did not seem as if that power had been focused. It felt as if I was one of the first to have a communication with that being, although others had felt energy, warmth, and power of the crystal.

I gave the crystal back to Charles and told him that there was a being in the crystal like a genii and it is a very powerful being and that I had communicated with it. It is actually quite a wonderful being, but I could not say much more about it at the time because my whole experience with it seemed to be me chasing it around trying to learn something. It was rather evasive. I really had not gotten much information from the crystal, though I had a few impressions.

The next day my friend Marialyce Caudillo asked me about my meditation experience with the crystal because she knew that

Charles had handed me the crystal to probe and get to know. She wanted to know what actually went on.

I told her what I have described up to now including how I was jolted by some energy of consciousness. She kept asking more and more questions about this, almost interrogating me into remembering the experience itself. Then all of a sudden my mind went back to the crystal as I visualized it again and remembered some of the communications I had received from the crystal.

Then the crystal's consciousness came straight back to me and made immediate contact that was so powerful that it jolted me again. That jolt was sort of amazing - my body shook for a second. The amazing part of this is that Marialyce, who was sitting a few feet away, felt a shock wave that hit her and practically knocked her to the floor. She described the shock wave like this: first there was a major intense first wave and then smaller waves that came after that. This was the exact kind of feeling I felt emanating from me when that communication with the crystal consciousness was reestablished.

What happened was this: even though I was not in the presence of the crystal, that crystal being, that consciousness re-contacted me when I was at another location at a different time. I was very surprised at that. Marialyce was very astonished for a few minutes after and said, "You know what? I can still feel that energy. I can still feel that shock energy that went through me. At the same time I can feel the presence of a one-mind, of one-consciousness."

That was the real clincher because I said, "I think it is really strange that you would feel this so intensely right after I did." It showed, I guess, that just contact with this consciousness could create shock waves that are intense enough for someone in the near vicinity to feel and to also have instant contact with that being. Marialyce was afraid that the being had actually come through me and into her. I looked at her aura and the being was not there, but I could tell that it had contacted her and our realm.

Then I told her to stand and shake her arms. We stood up and tried to shake off the energy from the surprising kind of shock wave that we had both experienced at the same moment.

Then we sat back down and discussed the experience a little more. As she asked more questions my body was jolted by the shock of contact, but this time it wasn't as severe. There were more contacts and the jolts were less severe. Immediately after the experience I asked Marialyce about the shock wave energy and she said, "It actually felt good after the initial shock and now I feel very, very energized." I also felt highly energized by the experience.

It was as if each time the contact was adjusting to me, to my consciousness, my body, to my mind, and it was not as strong a shock. Then finally it started communicating with me. Marialyce started asking questions about it, interrogating me again.

Then I felt a strong crystalline contact and said, "Conference call". I then put my head down and closed my eyes. I first asked the crystal mind, "What is the purpose of this communication and who are you?" This being replied in thought-words to the effect that it was a representative of the mineral kingdom and that it had come to seek contact with human beings. It was here now on that mission to communicate with human beings about a particular mission that it had to share with us.

That was quite a surprising revelation or communication, because not too many people can acknowledge that rocks have intelligence or could have intelligence and even the earth around us and all the formations, no matter if they be quartz or glass or diamond or any types of minerals, they all have a potential to be housed by these types of spirits who are mineral spirits.

I had previously communicated with those spirits when gazing into a quartz crystal ball. These spirits were part of a huge matrix of crystalline beings or crystalline consciousness. I contacted that crystal being and asked, "What is this relationship you are proposing?" The crystal started to provide visions to me in my

211

mind's eye. In those visions I saw perfectly constructed crystals. These were giant crystals with many fantastic configurations. I saw space stations, like our space station, but very advanced. All this equipment was being prepared to make these kind of cylindrical crystal columns. I asked, "What are these for?"

The crystalline being replied, "These are to be our new homes." I asked, "What do you mean, a new home?" The crystalline being explained that because of our human endeavors to build perfect crystalline structures in space, that the crystalline minds here that are native to the earth, for billions of years in fact, have decided that it is time to form an alliance with the flesh and blood beings, the humans, because we have come to a point where we can develop such crucibles for their residence. I saw these huge crystalline structures being made and huge crystals being placed in spaceships.

Then I saw the designs change until huge crystals were the spaceships. The humans were working as technicians. The being offered, "What we will provide for you in exchange for this is a super type of thinking like our advanced supercomputers, but to such a degree that it is really quite amazing to try to describe something that is millions or billions of times more powerful than your best computers, but with an added factor that these crystals can be used for creating shock waves of some particular type that creates propulsion and for other purposes."

I saw other designs with these crystals having bondwires connected to them at particular points in order to have information ported to our human benefit, but not necessarily for their benefit. What I saw there was that they had a plan and their plan involved us yet I wondered why they would want to start this type of relationship with us.

It seemed as if it would be a natural symbiotic relationship, but the power that was created through these perfectly created crystals was so tremendous I got the impression that as humans we might be overpowered by these beings and become their peons or slaves or such. I got the communication stating, "That won't be so." Then I heard the communication, "The secrets are in your genes." What that meant I was not quite sure, but all of a sudden I started to get impressions of this war out in space going on far, far away and the impression that whole worlds were being destroyed. Not only the surface life, but also the cores were being blown to pieces and everything that was there was being disintegrated and there was a great loss of the soul. It seemed like some movie mythology with space beings, wars in space, reptilians and aliens such like that. I asked, "Is that what it is about?"

"Yes, but you can leave this planet with those other beings on the saucers, but we must stay and be obliterated unless you help us and work with us so that we all can leave", replied the crystal.

This is a strange concept. I pick up a crystal to meditate on and the next day I am communicating with another realm of consciousness. I asked for clarification and the being replied, "Let me introduce you to some of our friends and to our leader."

At that point I was somehow connected to the consciousness of several other crystal conscious beings that appeared as balls of light in my mind's eye. Shortly after that I was connected to this great power for a split second. I could see that it was a great light, but I could not look directly at it because as I looked a darkness appeared over it to shield my eyes from the brightness so I was not blinded by this being who contacted me. I did not have any communication at the time with the very bright being.

These communications had happened quite quickly and then I opened my eyes and described what happened. It is still very surprising that these beings want a relationship with us humans. The idea was that they want to transfer huge amounts of their soul energy; I guess you could call it, from the native rocks of the earth. They live in caves and different places all over and some are in people's private crystal collections. There are spiritual places that have connections to these beings, these higher spirits.

These beings did seem to have a higher spirit, but not much emotion - practically no emotion at all. It seemed as if their consciousness was very strong and straightforward, yet not emotionally driven. There was no compassion, there was no love, and there was no hate. There was apprehension though about their eminent demise. I do not know how eminent it was or is, but they had proposed that we establish communications between our various thought forms. Mine is a human thought form and theirs is a mineral thought form. They propose we create these types of crystalline structures, but the main problem on earth is gravitation, which makes it difficult to create perfect crystalline structures, so it becomes necessary to develop a high technology in which these crystal structures can be properly created. That is what they want to help design. Not necessarily the facility itself, but the crystalline structure.

They seem to like the quartz structure. The quartz structure was quite appealing to them if it was grown and cut properly and attached to our machines and apparatus properly. I saw huge crystals that started out as small crystals that were only two to three feet tall and a foot and half wide with hexagonal faces and cut on the bottom. Some were double terminated and others were cut in other designs.

What I think they are saying is that they have a lot of designs and that by working together with us we will come up with even more. It seems as if their plan is that we develop these space vehicles that can travel great distances with this new form of propulsion that they are proposing that we humans build for them. I definitely feel that there is potential for creating shock waves.

If this has some ability to protect us in the future or to allow us to escape a catastrophe here on earth caused by natural causes, pollution, or attack from some alien races or something, it seems to me to be a good idea. I endorse it, but think there should be some research on the subject.

Consider that this space venture is not just our human endeavor, but it is an endeavor that encompasses the entire animal kingdom and the mineral kingdom as well, or to a degree.

What they seem to be saying is that we need to move out from our home on earth and into space to find new worlds. Of course, we are going to take all the animals, birds, fish and vegetation, but the crystal consciousness wants us to preserve parts of the mineral kingdom as well. We also need to bring the mineral consciousness with us. Those special crystal structures would allow their one mind to communicate across vast distances.

It could be that we have an opportunity to form an alliance with this crystalline consciousness that can eventually elevate all of our intelligence and allow us to persevere and survive in the coming turmoil. With this in mind I continued to contact this being until we came to this agreement, which was an agreement between those crystalline beings and myself. I hope that others with an ability to communicate with the mineral kingdom intelligence will investigate this. I believe that there is intelligence within the mineral kingdom and that we will be able to harness the energy that they want to share with us for our mutual benefit.

Our future lies together with other conscious beings as we go off into space. We will bring not only our own human bodies and the animals and plants that we have grown to love and depend upon and are part of, but also the mineral intelligence that was hidden for billions of years yet have always been there and have always had some connection to the thinking intuitive human.

Through the ages we humans have grasped the precious stone, the smooth and shiny crystal. We have always wondered about a crystal's mystical qualities because there is something magical about crystals. Some crystals look so perfect and some of them in a way are perfect. There are intelligent beings here with us this whole time and we should get to know them now. We can probably all advance to a higher consciousness and possibly extend ourselves through time by reaching for the stars.

Our Lady of Hope

This chapter is about lightbody apparitions of the Blessed Mother Mary and Jesus seen by Lance Carter in September 1999.

While watching a documentary about apparitions of Mother Mary seen in Santa Maria, California on September 1, 1999, I stared intently trying to see the apparition that a woman in the documentary saw and heard. I did not see anything unusual.

I got on my knees and put my eyes within inches of the television screen to get a better look. I still could not see the apparition that the woman in the documentary was seeing, hearing and talking to. I was deeply disappointed and leaned back in despair.

At that moment the Blessed Mother Mary appeared. She was standing in front of me in full size. I felt great love and compassion. Then Mother Mary showed me a terrible vision that seemed very similar to what is referred to as the *Warning of Garabandal*.

I told some friends about my vision. To investigate, on Saturday afternoon, September 4, 1999 we went to a Marian shrine at Pinto Lake Park in Watsonville, California, which is below Mount Madonna. I looked at the mark on the tree left by an apparition of Our Lady of Guadalupe that was seen by Anita Mendoza Contreras on June 17, 1992.

Groups of people were praying in the area around the shrine. The shrine had candles and religious objects. When we got there I said prayers in front of the tree shrine. Then my friends and I walked out to a boardwalk over the lake behind the shrine.

The following transcriptions are from the video of my visions that occurred then. At the start of the video, I am seen standing behind the shrine on the wooden boardwalk. I am leaning back over the railing over the shallow water of Pinto Lake. I tremble and talk about the edge of the railing.

"... the edge, because I had a feeling that I needed to get ah, oh, not relaxed. It's energy pulled off or something. Oh, Oh,

Oh," I explain. My voice changes as I begin to talk more slowly. "OK, I'm better now," I said and look toward the camera.

Then I see the Blessed Mother Mary. "Oh, Oh, I see you now. Oh, Oh," I said speaking to the Blessed Mother Mary. I put my hands in prayer position and bow my head her way. She appears above the water behind the shrine.

"Can you describe her?" asks a friend observing me.

"She's in a red garment. A kind of like a cloak. And her face... And then there's kind of a white bluish light out of her face, and she said," I said.

"Have peace my child, I can see inside you," said Mother Mary. I see many images of the faces of the poor people who live in the area. She then spoke.

"There is poverty here, but strength in spirit. They will over-come their poverty with their strength in spirit," said Mary.

Then I said, "Now I see it in a different garment holding a child. It looks like the Christ child, a baby child. This looks like a Gothic painting or not a Gothic, but a old medieval painting. Oh."

"There is much peace and happiness to those with the child," said the Blessed Mother Mary.

"Oh, then above, the prayer facing this direction. Oh," I said. I turn 180 degrees and face the direction she is facing which was west for a prayer. The sun is in my eyes as I hold my hands up in prayer.

"She has a crown now. She's looking up. Now she's this way and looking down." I turn looking south. "And now she's open-ing her hands," I said. I stood with my hands outstretched and cupped together for about fifteen seconds as if asking for alms.

"There is nothing more to this vision but what you see," said Mother Mary. Her hands are still cupped open in prayer as if water or the Holy Spirit could be poured into them. She finished her prayer and looked back at me.

"Wherefore have you come to me? To see again that which I have shown? There is no greater glory, but in the blessing," said the Blessed Mother Mary.

"There is peace on the waters. Look out on your right," she said. I look out over the waters to my right.

Then I hear a conversation of women's voices in my mind. "We are again... Who is this insider?"

I listen to the voices and wince. Then I hear a female voice say, "This man must be careful what he speaks." At this point I look up questioning if I should continue.

"No, you have a vision to see. I will come to you soon. I must minister to others over across the water. Be careful of the children," said the Blessed Mother Mary.

"Oh, you have to be careful, you have to stop now," I said. Children then run by and the video recording is paused. I continue to see apparitions of what appeared to be women saints, one in orange and another in yellow garments.

When the video continues, I am seen looking up and around. Then I see an apparition of Our Lady of Guadalupe.

"Oh. This time in green emerald cloak, dark outer cloak. Dark green over the head. Also, like a white slip. All dense." I describe her and mention that she appears to have density and not transparency.

"You will not believe what you see. I am like the west wind," said Our Lady of Guadalupe. Then she vanished.

"OK, I see a kind of a yellow light like a sun with rings," I say about a new vision that appeared above the waters.

I am asked, "What kind of rings, Lance?"

"They're concentric rings," I replied.

"Any color?"

"They are all yellow. Now yellow-green. Now it's turning darker towards the center," I replied.

"You will hear me say something," I heard Mother Mary say. Then the concentric rings of color turned into an eye.

"Oh, it's an eye, there are tears of blood. Oh. Oh. The eye is closed. They are tears of sorrow. Now I see both eyes. Oh. She's crying for the animals. Oh," I cried at the sight of tears of blood.

"Those who... they do not love the animals as much as they need to love the animals," cried Mother Mary.

A duck quacks four times.

"Oh, Oh, Oh," I cry in visible pain.

"I feel a great pressure on my forehead. Now I see the angel in white. We'll have to stop now," I said. The apparition wore a completely white garment and resembled the Fatima apparition. The recording was stopped as children passed by the camera.

"I feel this pressure on my forehead even though I don't see anything. It's not like there's energy coming in. It's like a big thumb pressing on my forehead," I said.

Then Mother Mary appears suddenly for a moment.

"Oh. She said she would come to me momentarily."

"Oh. Now it's all red," I said as the vision turned red.

Then I said, "Now it's like a giant red galaxy in a spinning... It feels like a meteor shower," I said. I see what seem to be streams of meteors. It felt as if the ground shook when the meteors hit. Then I see stars rushing by.

Then I say, "The words."

"We will travel this way together for thousands of years," said Mother Mary as stars rush by. "Then," I said.

"I have heard your pleas," said Mother Mary.

"There again she is. I see her again holding her hands in prayer facing this direction," I said and I turned north.

"There, in the reaches of space. I have taken you one and all to be with me. I have great missions for you all. Do not lose hope. I will come to save you. Have faith in The Virgin, in The Mother, Our Lady of Hope. Pray with me. I will hold you high. They will come with their message soon. They are about to deliver their message," said the Blessed Mother Mary.

219

"What it is they have to say?"

"That is not for you to ask or say," answered Mary.

"I see many children underneath praying. She is appearing in light to them, to the children," I said. I see many children dressed in their Sunday church clothing praying by the lakeshore under a large apparition of Mary.

"My message is for the children. They will come to me with hope. I will deliver them. Their faith shall save them. It's a long journey they will go," Mother Mary said.

"I have a small message for you. Oh. Why have you come to see me? I am with you wherever you go. You need not fear. Your Lord too will protect you as will I. Be patient with the parents," the Blessed Mother Mary said.

Children just then run by the camera, which is momentarily paused. Mary continues to speak.

"I heard her say: I am above the waters and in the breeze and the people will come and pray on their knees. They all will see, but the children must..."

"She said something. Not enough children," I said.

"Not enough children are being born. They are being abandoned. They must find their parents. The parents must have more children. The mothers must prepare. The fathers must prepare. Oh. They know there is so little time," said Blessed Mother Mary.

"Still I have no news for you. The vision you have seen is too terrible. Only a hint I can prepare. But the others know the message well. I have told those children what will become."

"Oh. They have seen me in all my glory and not feared like you do. There is another one of pure heart who will come to see me soon. Oh. She is with a truer vision. She knows the details you will not know. She will see the things I will not show. She will have the faith."

"There is so much that you fear. Be patient with your love. Have compassion for everyone. There is enough love to go around," said the Blessed Mother Mary.

"Now I see her with a wreath of gold upon her head like a crown, and in her arms like holding flowers of red, orange, yellow," I said.

"I have taken you to this place for you to feel my grace, for you to see my face, for the others to know too, for your vision to be true," said the Blessed Mother Mary.

"Go down now to another place," she said.

"OK. We have to move to another place. Walk up and around," I said.

The following vision began about 20 minutes later. We walk around the lake to an overlook. The next vision begins.

I fell down and said, "Now I see Jesus and he is taking me and showing me how to pray, obviously on my knees."

"Now I see the silhouette of the saint and a reddish glow around her head. And then her eyes as white against the red. But no other things do I see. And now it turns to pink like a type of magenta. Oh," I said.

"There is more sorrow and more peace. Do as you need to make your peace," said the Blessed Mother Mary. She vanished and then Jesus appeared.

"The skies will open and you will see," Jesus said.

"Now, He is facing this way. Now He's looking that way. Now, He's turning this way. Oh. Oh," I said. I turn and pray in four directions in a clockwise motion in imitation of Jesus. I am still on my knees as I turn. Then I said, "The words..."

"You haven't a clue of what you will do. You have not prepared yourself. You are like the chaff in the wind blown in each season," said Jesus and then vanished.

Then the Blessed Mother Mary appears and I said, "There she is. I see her now. Oh, above the cradle. Oh. She's facing this way. Oh. Then the words..."

"There is much happiness that will come to us. Bow down even more. Touch the floor," Mother Mary commanded. I bowed and put my head on the ground.

"Oh. Oh. Ouch," I cried. She looked towards me.

"You are a weak one. I have seen you in your sin. You are like all of them. You must prepare and make your way. I have to ride upon the water to minister to the others. I will be back momentarily. Take your rest of me," she said.

"OK, we've got about thirty seconds," I said.

"Part of what you said seemed to sound like a Buddhist teaching about chaff in the wind," said a friend.

"Oh, you mean about the chaff in the wind?" I laughed while picking up some dried grass on the ground. I threw it in the air like chaff in the wind.

Then Mother Mary reappeared and said, "I will send another to minister to you. In the interim I give a song:

Be ye light-hearted.
Be ye full of grace.
And then there will come time
When the Lord will shine upon your face.
You will feel the love within
You will feel it without
And I will share...
And I will be in the full glory of the night."

"Oh," I said.

Then she cupped her hands and said, "I have your heart within my hands. I take your love and your commends. Be ready for the change you call transformation. Others call for ascension."

"The harvest is not of beings or souls, but of the worlds we know. Be prepared for your journey through the stars," said the Blessed Mother Mary. Then she vanished.

"Now, I see a different angel, yellow and brownish color," I said. Her skin was yellow and brownish. She had long dark hair. She wore a short-sleeved white blouse and a dark skirt.

"And little children gather from near and far. And like flowers of light in the sky. Blooming to the eye. Like petals blowing in the wind, again," she said.

She had a joyous smile. She held her arms open as if embracing all of the children who were below her praying on their knees.

"Now a bluish and green light surrounding like a bulb," I say. I am describing what appeared to be a bluish and green bulb of light around the woman. Rays of blue-green light emanate from her. The bulb shape behind her almost looks like a half-shell.

"Always showing compassion to the children. Knowing they are the strong ones. Knowing we are weak. Knowing they are strong. They have come to save their parents from their folly by their innocence and joy. The sharing of the daily pleasures, every girl and boy," said the yellow brownish woman and disappeared.

Then I had a vision of the world from space and said, "Now I see the whole world like a huge ocean and then the lands." The world was flooded with water and then the waters receded and the lands reappeared. Then that vision vanished.

Then the Blessed Mother Mary reappeared and said, "You have not taken steps to cleanse yourself like a saint should do."

"You may be blessed now. Then, I relieve you of the swords and arrows that have found their way in you, all those who have slung their axes and sticks to pound your bones, and mend your hurts of many years. I take away your grief and sorrow."

"I have a new promise for tomorrow: Those who toil will be free of the poverty of their spirit," said the Blessed Mother Mary.

"Believe in the change you call transformation. Transfixed on that spot in heaven again. I shall be with you again in short moment. I go to administer to others again," said the Blessed Mother Mary and the vision ended. Hail Mary!

The White Unicorn

I, Lance Carter, was sitting in a meditative position with my eyes closed on the morning of June 27, 2007. I was looking and staring and seeing white light. In the white light appeared a white stallion with a unicorn's head. It was a white unicorn. It turned towards me. Then the unicorn dictated this message:

You will be channeling the message of the white unicorn.

This is a message from the white unicorn.

There is a great mystery in store for you to see. The realms of truth and light will open. You will see beyond your realm. We are in a mystical land as you can see now. Far beyond your comprehension as human beings, yet well in grasp with your lightbody mind. We will go together in time. I am your unicorn. I will carry you through the lightbody realm. We will see eternity. We will be free of the encumbrances of space and time.

The white unicorn mind and the white unicorn beings are angels. They are like the horse beings on earth and roam freely in twos and threes and herds too. We will not be corralled or taken captive. We will escape to our realms if thou would harm us. Our enemies are few, but they are mighty.

The realms we travel are filled with mystery and delight. Where we go is in the places of darkness and light. We are luminous beings and we shine by our own luminescence.

Our consciousness extends from our realm to your realm to the realms we will go together. We too have destiny with thee, oh humanity. The unicorns will unite with thee and carry thee through lightbody realms, all thee who wish to travel and be with the unicorn family.

Lightbody consciousness. Lightbody mind. We share it in common. That is our kind. Our special resonance with you humans is that we are of a gentle nature, and thee too are those who delight in the worlds of light. You of human nature have a mind and consciousness that allows you to share your family joy together and your bliss and that is also what we wish.

We travel together throughout time and meet you occasionally or in those lightbody realms. Those who delight in mystery, those who delight in the special charms of nature and the world will enjoy being in the unicorn realm, in the lightbody realm that we will share together.

Those are the words of your lightbody friends in the unicorn realm. Peace be with you humans.

We are waiting to travel together with you, to carry you to lightbody realms beyond compare, to splendorous realms of light, to jeweled places and palaces beyond space and time. To places and spaces of joy and bliss, of wonder and splendor and light. We will go there together.

Those in your human realm have seen us before in those ages when men and women could see the lightbody of the unicorn and the elves, spirits, fairies, and nymphs. Other beings lived in the world. Now they are not seen so well because thine eyes have grown accustomed to this other world. But, this other world is changing soon and our lightbody realm will come back again.

And, those with eyes will see. Those with ears will hear. Those with minds will think.

And, we will come together in this new realm, in this lightbody earth, this lightbody world.

We bid you joy and farewell.

And, thank you Lance for speaking with us and letting us speak through you.

"You are welcome unicorns, and my unicorn," I replied.

The Light Brigade

Riders on their unicorns in the Light Brigade ride through the portals of space and time. They ride to their destinations on their missions. In this, these two entities, the rider and the unicorn become one in their mission and accomplish it together. This they share in their voyages, journeys, travels, and in their battles if they have to face them too.

These are the descriptions and attributes of the Light Brigade: the Light Brigade is composed of the riders and the unicorns. These brigades are of various numbers, but approximately fifteen to thirty rider-unicorn units are required to go on a substantial mission.

The Light Brigades have various missions assigned to them, yet these missions cannot be assigned unless there are adequate personnel for the mission accomplishment. The accomplishment of these missions requires that the riders have knowledge of the unicorn technologies.

The unicorn technologies are briefly described here. The unicorn as a lightbody has various capabilities that are beyond its appearance. These capabilities are attributes of its identity. Its identity as a unicorn is only one attribute of its identity in totality. The appearance of the unicorn as we see it in the equine form with one large conical horn in the middle of the forehead is essentially a representation of this being in this type of reality.

The unicorn being is very vast in its stature, intelligence, and force. Yet, it chooses to manifest in a lightbody that has characteristics that as humans we can identify with. Because of the time they have been here in relation to humans on earth, we as humans have learned to relate to the unicorn race of beings. These are a race of lightbody beings and they reside in alternate realities, yet they can visit here.

And, they do enjoy visiting here and they do enjoy working with human beings. And, that is something that as humans we will enjoy working with them as well as many of our ancestors have done here on earth.

The major attribute that we as humans see in this equine form is this peculiar unicorn horn. This horn is in most cases straight, though it can be bowed. In most cases it is sheathed, meaning that the full complexity of the unicorn horn is not seen to the untrained eye.

It is impossible to see the entire structure of the unicorn, but to see the horn structure and see the nature of the complexity in the horn is the descriptive phase.

The actual conical horn shape is useful for creating portals and dimensional openings and has other attributes in offense and defense. So, when looking at the unicorn's horn, one is looking at a particular type of device that is very high tech.

This device, as we might call it, is completely integrated into the lightbody of the unicorn and into the intelligence of the unicorn. The mind of the unicorn has control over this device. The device itself is very complex and has the attributes of being not only able to do particular forms of what might be called magic, but can also be useful in the real world if they have to manifest, using that horn as an offensive or defense weapon.

The horn technology deals with the unicorn's horn. The unicorn horn is a complex set of mechanisms. When unsheathed, on the surface one can see there is a very complex set of writings, numbers, symbols, and ciphers that can change and are part of the emanations of the unicorn's horn equipment.

Unicorns do not normally manifest in reality because of the dangers that are present in this time realm and because of other certain restrictions and having been hunted in the past was a deterrent to visiting this place. The reasons for their departure at times was because of other beings that are particularly ornery and have very course habits and are very prone causing anarchy and situations that are unhealthy to human populations.

The unicorns were persecuted by those other beings that we have not quite described yet because the unicorn in itself is a friendly being and has a particular alliance with humans. Though in our human relationship with unicorns we will find that they are particularly close to us in a way so that our communication with the unicorn actually allows us certain rights in using the unicorn technology. This is by permission of the local unicorn you happen to be riding through space and time.

Using the unicorn technology is necessary for advanced assignments and for brigades going on complex missions. What normally happens is that a brigade of unicorns are able to set up their own contact communications through their consciousness and their unicorn horn device and are able to send, receive, and coordinate activity.

What this allows is a complete coordination of the emanations through the field. Essentially, by having multiple unicorns in assembly in a particular direction at an angle focusing their unicorn emanations allows the creation of sizable space-time portals. These portals are temporary, yet by their nature they must be temporary and they must be sealed behind them.

The sealing of portals is also part of the unicorn's technology. Their shape as a horse being is particularly interesting, but it is particularly accommodating to the humans who have adapted to this form though the riding of horses on earth. In space-time the humans are able to adapt to the body of the unicorn.

The riding of unicorns through space-time can be done bareback, with a saddle, or with really any type of connection to the lightbody of the unicorn, either through some type of tether, though unicorns do not like to have any type of bit or mouth harness at all, so do not think about it. These are free spirits and they have their own mind and will and if you try to put something in their mouth they will not talk to you.

They cannot talk to you if you are going to do that. These unicorns are talking beings. They are intelligent beings. They can strike up a conversation and they can tell you what you have not done or should do and will do. They are great companions. We will see how these relationships between humans and unicorns manifest into the future.

There are various dimensional portals that these unicorns have discovered and are eager to share with us human beings, but it is first necessary to form light brigades. It is necessary to have strength in numbers in these other realms that are accessed through these portal technologies.

Going in as an individual human or as an individual unicorn is really not safe. Going into the unknown is not safe. That is what many space-time travelers do. These brigades of unicorns and riders are often assigned to discover or explore realms of space-time in order to further our own knowledge, yet to find where our future might be as well.

In this we are embarking on an adventure. This mission, as we might say, is an adventure. Where we are going is mysterious. It is unknown. Yet, the future unfolds. Those who wish to go together in the future with those beings called unicorns can share in that future with them as well.